Navigating Through A Strange Land

A Book for Brain Tumor Patients and Their Families

Navigating Through A Strange Land

A Book for Brain Tumor Patients and Their Families

Tricia Ann Roloff

Indigo Press

Library of Congress Cataloging-in-Publication Data

Navigating through a strange land : a book for brain tumor patients
  and their families / [edited by] Tricia Ann Roloff
      p. cm.
  Includes bibliographical references and index,
  ISBN 0-9641214-1-7 (pbk.)
1. Brain--Cancer--Popular works. 2. Brain--Cancer--Psychological aspects. 3. Brain--
Cancer--Patients--Family relationships.
I. Roloff, Tricia Ann, 1958-
RC280.B7N38   1994
362.1'9699481--dc20   94-25863
                                                                          CIP

    Design and typesetting: Diane Spencer Hume
    The editor is grateful for permission to reprint the following copyrighted materials:
    Letter portion of "Jamie's story" from "To Live Until We Say Goodbye," by Elizabeth Kubler-
Ross and Mal Warshaw. Copyright © 1978 by Ross Medical Associates, S.C. and Mal
Warshaw. Used by permission of Prentice-Hall, a division of Simon & Schuster.
    "Hope" by William Buchholz. Copyright © 1990, by the Journal of the American
Medical Association. Used with the permission of JAMA (JAMA, 1990;263:2357-2358).
    Richard Hail's story, originally published in Search, copyright © 1987 National Brain
Tumor Foundation, and Richard Hail. Used with permission by NBTF and Richard Hail.
    Norman Kornsand's story, originally published in Search, copyright © 1988 National
Brain Tumor Foundation, and Norman Kornsand. Used with permission by NBTF and Norman
Kornsand.
    Sections from the International Herald Tribune Weekend Edition article "Modern
Fiction on the Couch," by Anatole Broyard, Jan 17, 1986. Copyright © 1986 by The New
York Times Company. Reprinted by permission.
    Cover art: oil on canvas titled Letaba I, copyright © 1988, by Thirza Kotzen
    Cartoon on page 211 by David Sypress, copyright © 1989
    All other illustrations: original color pencil sketches by Tricia Roloff, copyright
© 1982, 1992
    Printed in the U.S.A. by Gilliland Printing, Inc.

indigo press
New Address:
P.O. Box 968
West Fork, AR 72774-0968
501-839-3944

2nd Printing, January 1997

This book is dedicated to the authors who made it happen. They gave their time and dedication without compensation to help others; and that is the most noble of all gifts.

Creative people do not try to run from their feelings of non-being, but by encountering and wrestling it, force it to produce being. They knock on silence for an answering machine, they pursue meaninglessness until they can force it to mean.

—Rollo May, from *The Courage to Create*

Contents

Foreword x
Preface xii
Acknowledgments xiv

Part One
Chapter One: Exploring the Terrain 3
    An Overview of Brain Tumors; Who to Look to For Help
    During Treatment and Recovery

Part Two
Chapter Two: Patients Tell How They Cope 23
    Surround Yourself with Those You Love 25
        Kristan Elizabeth Randolf (Glioblastoma Multiforme)
    A Happy Ending After a Long and
    Confusing Journey 29
        Laura Santi (Ganglioneuroma)
    Healing Is a Lifelong Process 38
        Marie Beckerman (Meningioma)
    A 20-Year Survivor: Her Story and Reflections 44
        Kris Simonsen (Craniopharyngioma)
    I Could Now Do All the Things I Dreamed About 63
        Norman Kornsand (Glioblastoma)
    Experimenting with RU 486 67
        Fume Takano (Meningioma)
    Life is Like Climbing a Mountain 72
        Chris Kuchera (Astrocytoma)
    Friends Pleaded with Me to
    Go to the Doctor 76
        Julie Arlinghaus (Juvenile Pilocytic Astrocytoma)

It's a Cruel, Crazy, Beautiful World.............................. 81
    Chris de Jong (Glioblastoma Multiforme)
What it Means To be Human 99
    Tricia Roloff (Pituitary Adenoma)

Chapter Three: Family Members Tell Their Stories 113
    I No Longer Fear Death... 115
        Linda's Story
    May His Dream Someday Come True....................... 122
        Bonnie Feldman
    We Realized a Lot of Things Too Late 132
        Dr. Darryl Forstner (alias)
    I Could Hardly Say the Words:
    My Daughter Has Cancer 140
        Richard Hail
    Her Love Still Abides 143
        Harry Smith

Chapter Four: Professional Caregivers 153
    Modern Fiction on the Couch:
    An Interview With a Retired Psychoanalyst 155
        Anatole Broyard, former book reviewer, New York *Times*
    Focus on the Things You Can Control 159
        Dr. Charles Wilson, Professor and former Chairman,
        Department of Neurosurgery, University of Califor-
        nia, San Francisco; Director, Brain Tumor Research
        Center

    Every Tumor Has a Brain:
    Assessing Neurological Changes. 167
        Dr. John Walker, Assistant Professor of Neuro-psychol-
        ogy, Department of Neurology, University of Califor-
        nia, San Francisco

What About Our Faith?
Reflections of a Hospital Chaplain 177
    Reverend Karyn Gladson, Director of Pastoral Care,
    Long Beach Memorial Medical Center, Long Beach, CA
A Zen Approach 188
    Debra Jan Bibel, Ph.D.
Hope Is a Prescription: One Doctor's Analysis 189
    Dr. William Buchholz, private practice, Los Altos, CA
The Patient and the Physician
Have to Fight Together 198
    Dr. Nicholas de Tribolet, Chairman of Neurosurgery,
    University Hospital, Lausanne, Switzerland

Chapter Five: An Afterward 201
Never Underestimate Yourself

Part Three
Chapter Six: Resources 207
    Tumors and Treatment 212
    Personal Contact 214
    Brain Tumor Foundations and Associations 214
    Other Services and Information 218
    Legal and Financial Planning 223
    Reading List 225

Index 231

Foreword

At some time in our lives most of us face a personal medical challenge whether for ourselves or, while in support of a loved one. We manage these challenges the best we can at the time—trying to understand and make sense of what is happening and trying to work with our health care providers for the best possible results. The most helpful support during this time often comes from a personal story or experience shared by someone who has also lived through the same challenge. The opportunity to learn from what other people have learned through their experiences and gained from the challenges is invaluable.

This book provides that invaluable opportunity for patients, families and caregivers living with a brain tumor diagnosis. Ms. Roloff has gathered a range of individual experiences with brain tumors—from people who face this diagnosis, family members who have provided support and professional caregivers who work with brain tumor patients. These personal stories are not intended to show a "right" or "wrong" way to manage living with a brain tumor. In fact, it is reassuring that no two stories are exactly the same. Rather, the stories convey the individual's experience and the shared universal concerns —personal fears, small victories and disappointments and the uncertainties of living with a brain tumor.

The stories are usefully designated by type of brain tumor and include both benign and malignant diagnoses. The stories include first-person accounts of treatment and recovery, experimentation with a controversial drug in clinical trial and what steps people took to participate in their own health care decisions. There are the perspectives of family members on the death of parents and children and the self-help advice and observations of health care professionals.

In addition, Ms. Roloff provides practical information to assist in the understanding of brain tumors, encouragement for individuals to be assertive about their personal wants and needs in the delivery of their health care, coping techniques including the use of art, advice for financial and legal planning and a generous section of resources (organizations, books, pamphlets, support groups and professional contacts).

This book can help empower anyone facing the challenge of a brain tumor with the wisdom, dignity and knowledge of shared experiences.

Tracy Cosgrove, M.L.I.S.
Director, Planetree Health Resource Center
San Francisco, CA.

Preface

Months after I had surgery in 1984, I came upon a small eight-page booklet (no longer in print) that described in a few paragraphs pituitary tumors and common problems associated with them. I found that booklet very comforting; I clung to it in fact, for several months, until I could come to grips with what had happened.

I believe people do rebound pretty well from most things, given time. That time though may be longer for one person than another. And it seems there are natural recurrences of what I call 'reflective grief' of the event throughout a person's lifetime. But, I also think it's about time that people be given credit for the strengths they do show when faced with such a situation. There seems to be so much focus on what's wrong with people.

From 1987-1989 I worked as editor for the National Brain Tumor Foundation and helped put together their newsletter. This book is somewhat an extension of what we did there; highlighting people's experiences. At the same time I was hired by the University of California, San Francisco and worked for seven years in an administrative position in a research lab, in addition to continuing my free-lance writing business on the side.

I worked on many scientific manuscripts for publication. Research is a slow process, and results for the understanding and treatment of illnesses take many, many years. Because research is so slow in getting answers (although in the end it provides the only significant answers), it's even more important that there be emotional support for people, because there are no quick fixes.

I have always believed that truth can only be expressed as a result of personal experience, and thus made a goal to put together a text which reflected the truths of a brain tumor diagnosis. I believe I have accomplished what I set out to do: I have given you stories of triumph, stories of death, stories of pain and stories of gratitude. There were no great heroics, only the day to day realities. And that is the truth of it.

About the book itself. The cover art is an oil on canvas done by my friend and former university art professor, Thirza (Gute) Kotzen. She lives in London with her husband and exhibits in Europe and Johannesburg, South Africa, her hometown. The title of the book came to mind as I looked at a picture of this painting and reflected on how I myself was literally in a foreign land when I suspected something was wrong with me.

Drawing was my way of coping with a lot of strange feelings then. I have included some of these drawings at the front of each chapter. To look at them now, after all these years, certainly reminds me of my ordeal with the tumor; but equally they fill me with joy. They were done in Seville, Segovia, Toledo, and Madrid, Spain.

Acknowledgments

There are many people I wish to thank. First and foremost , I thank Sharon Lamb, R.N. for her unswerving support of all my efforts over the years. Her work and genuine concern are an inspiration to all who know her. More recently, Dr. Maribelle Leavitt whom I met at the beginning of this project and who has also been a positive influence. Dr. Charles Wilson for his initial interest in this publication which gave me the confidence to pursue it. To Kris Simonsen, my dear friend, whose honesty and determination were the initial inspiration for this writing, and who also helped with important editorial and design suggestions in the final draft . To other staff at the University of California, San Francisco who have offered continuing encouragement and advice. Most notably, my former colleagues Charlene Bayles, Debra Jan Bibel, and Jane Leong. To my sister Sue, and my friend Lisa Peterson who told me I had to finish it when I felt like quitting. To Jeff Fink for his love and for critiquing and editing parts of the book. A heartfelt thanks to Dr. Robert West of International Scholars Publications for invaluable publishing assistance. A very special thanks to Gute. And thank you, of course, to my parents, whose love sustains me.

Part One

Chapter One

Exploring the Terrain

Navigating Through a Strange Land

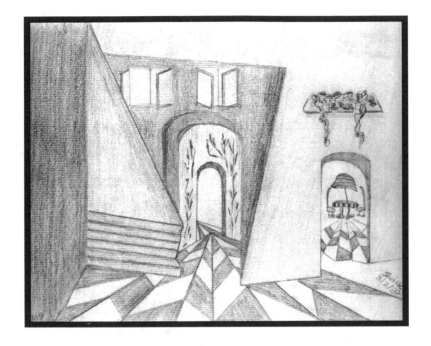

Exploring the Terrain

Something's Just Not Right

For a time you will be traveling through a land that is foreign to you. Many have been there before you, although their landscape will look a little different than yours. May this book help familiarize you with some of the terrain.

Dealing with the diagnosis of a brain tumor is tough. It's not like a broken arm, or another part of your body that you can look at and say, "OK just five weeks and we'll be back to new, maybe even a little stronger." It's more like a heart attack, where a person feels that a part of their very being has been disturbed - the part that pumps life, that hurts when things feel bad, that breaks when a love affair ends.

With something in the brain, we fear our very mind will start slipping away. Depending on where the tumor is located, areas that control motor function, memory, as well as orientation, balance, coordination, speech, sight, and chemistry can easily be effected, either temporarily or permanently. This fact alone makes this diagnosis particularly scary, because sound intellectual function is what allows us to do our jobs, raise our families, and create our own special life.

Navigating Through a Strange Land

Not one disease, but many

Brain tumors occur in a variety of ways, and it is now believed that they are the result of not just one disease, but many. This presents researchers and physicians with a difficult task in finding the cause(s) and in determining the perfect treatment(s).

Every year approximately 20,000 primary brain tumors are diagnosed and another approximately 40,000 or maybe more travel to the brain from other parts of the body (metastasize). Diagnoses in people 65 and older has increased significantly. Women made up 46% of new brain tumor patients in 1992, although its the largest cause of cancer death in men 15-35, and the second most common cause of cancer death in children behind Leukemia.

Astrocytomas, the most commonly diagnosed tumors are graded I-IV depending on their aggressiveness. At stage IV astrocytomas are called glioblastomas. At this stage they are considered highly malignant and very difficult to treat. There is variance, however, in how these particular tumors are categorized, depending on where you are being treated. They are all serious though, despite what they are called.

Some tumors are noncancerous [benign], like meningiomas, and pituitary tumors. These are generally slow growing, and are often noticed only when they effect another part of the brain, like eyesight, coordination, or the hormone system. Terms like slow growing, and benign, however, are considered by some to be misleading, because all tumors within the brain have the potential of being life-threatening if not treated.

Some tumors start growing in adulthood, while others like craniopharyngioma, medulablastoma and brain stem gliomas often start in childhood. Cancer in children, of course, is the most difficult to understand. It is horribly traumatic for parents.

Move over, I'm a brain tumor!

Brain tumors are generally described as 'a cancer," which means that the cells keep dividing and multiplying, instead of stopping at a certain point. Because the tumor is in your brain and there is only so much space there, these cells push themselves upon and into vital structures within the different lobes or sections of the brain.

Some sections, like the frontal lobe, affect memory. The hypothalamus is the seat of our moods. Unlike an arm or a leg, though, our brain controls our thoughts and behavior, and a tumor can cause disruption in any one of these areas. That is why when a patient gets angry, depressed or violent, it may just as easily be caused by the physical placement of the tumor.

So brain tumors are unique because while we classify them as a 'cancer', they are really a neurological problem; they affect us neurologically, or in the case of pituitary tumors, hormonally. Because we know a fair amount about the brain, it is somewhat predictable to state upon location of the tumor, how and what it may affect.

Because 'cancer' is so pervasive there is plenty of ruminating on its causes: is it genetic or our environment; philosophically, is it a manifestation of an ill society at large; or metaphysically, is it an expression of our deepest personal conflicts brought to physical form? As for brain tumor disease, there is no evidence for any one cause. With the recent advances in molecular biology, researchers are trying to determine if there are genetic causes for the various tumors. And there is some real progress on this front. But for now, "Why do I have a brain tumor?" is not medically answerable.

No rhyme or reason

Some brain tumors are curable immediately by operation, or controlled throughout life by drugs, while some brain tumors after treatment go into remission for very long periods of time and then return, for no apparent reason. Some people live forever, even after a bad diagnosis from their physician, with no lingering problems, while others need to adjust their routines to accommodate new problems. Some people will die even when things seem to be going well. There seems to be no rhyme or reason to the course a brain tumor will take, or a reliable way to predict its outcome. In a way, this unpredictability is good news, because it means that for each person there is a chance, even if statistics say otherwise.

Current treatment for brain tumors include surgery and/or any combination of chemotherapy (drug therapy) and radiation, depending on the tumor type and degree of operability. If the 'tentacles' so to speak of a tumor have spread into vital structures, the surgeon may decide it's too dangerous to try to get the whole thing. And thus, you will need to have radiation or chemotherapy. Also, they can never be sure if they got all remaining cells, even if they got most of the tumor; some cells float away. So, there are several reasons for applying both treatments, rather than just one.

The newest treatment is the gamma knife, a technique that uses magnetic resonance (MR) and computer tomography (CT) guidance to map the exact location of the tumor and using complex physics beams the tumor with radiation. This has proved very successful for *certain* cases, but not all. Its advantage is that a patient is put into a tubelike cylinder, like an MRI machine, and treated without having to undergo surgery. It is used mainly on small tumors, because it destroys normal tissue, and therefore cannot be used on larger areas in the brain.

Navigating Through a Strange Land

Dealing with professionals

When diagnosed it is important to get several opinions (unless it is an emergency) and to investigate all of your options. This is your right. Your first loyalty is to yourself, not one institution, or one particular physician. In determining who will treat you one guideline to follow is the experience of the physician. Most neurosurgeons focus on the particular area that interests them. They specialize and become an expert in that area. Some even specialize in a particular tumor type. Asking respected physicians who they would go to if they had a brain tumor is a good start.

While many may be in private practice, many work in large university settings where they can do research along with their clinical practice. But large hospitals are more bureaucratic and may be less personal than, say, a community hospital. This is the nature of the beast. Therefore, if you are dealing with a large hospital, the first thing you should do is to select the person who will be coordinating events during your stay. This can be a nurse, social worker, or someone who can help you outline and understand your course of treatment, care, and later rehabilitation. Many people feel lost in a setting like this (understandably) and so feel they are the ones who are responsible for this coordination. This doesn't have to be. You can make

the necessary decisions and still leave the coordination to someone else. This will alleviate unnecessary
anxiety.

This is also a good time to organize your finances.
Follow the Boy Scout's motto, "Be Prepared." Talk with
your health insurance agent, and the financial planning
office of the hospital to make sure you understand exactly what your obligations will be, if any. This will
allow you time if you need to obtain loans or other help.

A lawyer who does estate planning might also be
someone you want to talk with. A comprehensive financial plan (estate plan) is important if you have a sizeable
estate and are truly concerned with the outcome of a
surgery or treatment.

It is estimated that only 54% of the population makes
a formal estate plan, and this causes many misunderstandings among family members. An estate plan consists
mainly of a will, or the popular living trust, as the center-
piece, and the following documents: Health care power
of attorney; financial power of attorney; nomination of
conservator; letter of instruction; a pour over will (with a
living trust); and property agreement (between a husband and wife).

Although the thought of it is initially uncomfortable,
taking care of these matters usually makes people feel
more at peace; it's one less thing to worry about. One
lawyer I consulted speculated the reason that people don't

do plans, is that they're afraid to face all their unrealized dreams. He commented that "what people don't realize is that we all only have time for so many things in life and so all our dreams get trickled down through a funnel into which only a few things can pass. And that's OK." How nicely put!

Who to look to for help

Neuroscience nurses and clinic staff

While you are staying in the hospital and during your recovery afterwards, there are several people you can turn to for help. A good caring nurse on your side and by your side can be one of your greatest assets while going through the medical system. Nurses have a lot of knowledge and experience. They will often take the time to talk with you and direct you if your physician is too busy to do so. Not all physicians are comfortable with or have the time to devote to the emotional needs of patients and sometimes this has to be accepted. But that doesn't mean that there is no one to help you.

Years after my surgery, while working for the National Brain Tumor Foundation, I met Sharon Lamb, R.N, who is vice president of the Foundation. She has helped me in many ways over the years and I only wish I had known her at the time of my surgery. Many patients treated at the University of California, San Francisco (UCSF) feel that she and the other nurses and staff have been their saviors and no less.

Here's another example. When Peter Farbach of Washington D.C. was treated for a brain tumor it was his first experience in any hospital. He writes, "For your next edition, how about a story describing the impact of nurse practitioner, Margaret Fiore, on my life. When I was struggling to save my identity and self-esteem in the spiritual darkness of that alien medical world, she brought me a window of light and hope, by treating me one-to-one as a person, rather than just another chart-with-symptoms patient in a dressed-in-white bureaucracy. She stayed in the operating room during all four of my craniotomies, though not a surgical nurse herself. Now she is coordinator of our support group here in the District. Margaret recently told me her favorite prayer - "God, make me a window for your light to shine through." I cherish and respect her selfless way of being that window for me and other people with brain tumors."

Personally, my greatest solace during my hospital experience was Shirley, a clinic administrative assistant, who spent countless hours calming my nerves. She was my only hospital-related outlet then, and I still think of her with great affection and gratitude.

Navigating Through a Strange Land

Social workers

Another valuable resource would be the social worker. Most hospitals have clinical social workers on staff. Some specialize in the neurooncology area while others are generalized. This depends on the size and staffing of the hospital. Clinical social workers can be tremendously helpful because they are exposed daily to the needs of patients. They understand the webwork of social services provided by cities and counties, understand issues of disability and vocational and rehab training. They are a resource center and should be consulted if available.

Chaplains

Hospitals also have chaplains. In fact, one of the best books I've read on loss and recovery was written by a hospital chaplain. Her name is Ann Kaiser Sterns and her book is *Living Through Personal Crisis*. I highly recommend this book.

Therapists

After you are through the initial treatment phases, psychologists and other therapists can have enormous value. The two that I would recommend as a beginning are a neuropsychologist and a family counselor.

A neuropsychologist will help define your neurological functioning, deficits, and strengths. Tests will be taken to determine specific task oriented comprehension and abilities. This will help you to understand which symptoms are caused by the brain tumor, and which ones are not. Memory problems are a good example. This testing can also help determine which skills you will be able to use in the future, which can be redeveloped in rehabilitation and which cannot. For some of you this might mean a change of jobs or careers, and vocational training or other therapy, such as speech therapy will be recommended. Disability claims also require written documentation. Given the complexity of the brain, neuropsychologists can help you immensely. Dr. Walker will discuss this later in the book.

Secondly, Marriage and Family Counselors (MFCC) are trained therapists who focus on your interpersonal relationships. Just as the moon effects the tides, as families we are bound into unified systems. Clearly what affects one family member affects and changes the interactions of all family members.

How can I develop good coping strategies? How can I help my family understand me? Why do I feel depressed? Is there something I can do about it? A good therapist can help you work through these issues, individually or with your family.

In addition, since these therapists specialize in 'families dynamics' they understand on a deeper level how our original interactions affect how we relate to others. We tend to adopt a particular role in our family and this role gets played out in many of our interactions. It may also predict how we will handle our illness. Families are usually the least equipped to handle the psychological aspects of a medical problem when it is *their* loved one, and many hurt feelings arise out of the misunderstandings that occur in this situation. If this is the case with you and your family don't be ashamed to ask for outside help.

Don't be afraid to be choosy

There are many types of therapy and therapists: There is psychotherapy, psychoanalysis, counselors, art therapists, M.A.'s, Ph.D's, etc. Titles from prestigious institutions are not necessary here; what is necessary is someone who makes you feel important and supported so that you can work on the issues that brought you to therapy. There is a lot of damage done by people who just apply a 'standard routine' to any problem, or who likewise come across as judgemental and cold. This is *not* just any problem, and you deserve someone who is truly there for you. Ask for referrals from friends. A good therapist can be a lifesaver and life-changer. I know many people who have felt this way. Also, therapy doesn't have to be a life long process. Short term therapy directed at a specific concern is usually all that is needed; a bridge over a troubled patch, or a way to have someone help direct events in a positive direction, rather than overwhelm you.

Your friends and fellow brain tumor patients

Last, but most important, your greatest source of strength may come from your friends and from others who have been down the road before you. Many people who go to a support group find that they instantly bond with others going through the same thing; the usual barriers to communication are absent and an open and honest dialogue is immediately established. Discussions in these meetings center around both the frustrations and the triumphs of the day. Many friendships form because it is a place where people can just be themselves, share ideas, find humor in their predicament, and so forth.

There are those who say of themselves, "well I'm a private person, I'm better if I handle it alone;" or, "I tried that and it doesn't work for me." And that's OK: like everything else, these kinds of meetings are not for everyone. But, I believe there are two instances where it can really help.

The first is in the acute stage of the illness; right after diagnosis or surgery or other treatment. A group run by a professional can help to answer many of the medical questions as well as give you hope by seeing others who have made it through. After the initial trauma period has ended, then other methods may work better for you, such as individual therapy, in which you can get help without sacrificing personal privacy, or a phone conversation with one of the former patient volunteers.

The second situation is if you are single and have no other primary support person like a spouse or relative close by available to help you. Doing everything yourself will overwhelm you with stress.

Navigating Through a Strange Land

If you have a good marriage or relationship where the other person is emotionally available and helps with the day to day needs, this will take a great burden off of you. However, being a caretaker is difficult if it extends for a long period of time. It's important to evaluate how much you can realistically expect of any one person, even if they love you. Over the long haul family and friends are what hold you together, but also be aware that professionals can help you.

In preparing this book I wanted to express hope for those diagnosed with this disease, as there is still a belief that anyone diagnosed with a brain tumor is going to die. This is simply not true. I know this through my own experience, and my work with the National Brain Tumor Foundation for the past seven years. In fact, every person I talked with during the writing of this book knew of someone who has had a brain tumor. It is much more common than we think. As with every disease some will die, and these people must be helped to die with dignity and grace. But there are many people who survive and live good lives in spite of their brain tumor experience.

At the same time, there are some problems. Along with the sometimes difficult search for the 'best treatment', there are the psychological and physical changes that can occur because of the tumor. These have mainly to do with changes in mental functioning and the emotional dilemmas that families and individuals face. Mental changes are a little easier to determine given the testing that is available. Emotional dilemmas are harder to identify; ranging from denial of family members, to simply not knowing how to cope. The personal stories that make up this book represent a realistic range of experiences and issues faced by brain tumor patients. You will see how very differently each person is affected.

Having access to appropriate information is the first step in dealing with the many issues that you will be faced with. If you have come across this book first, you should know that there are numerous foundations and associations in the United States and Canada who can help you. These people can provide you with information on support groups, treatments, physician referrals and more in depth medical information. I could not begin to replicate all of their work. My main concern is to address the psychological issues rather than compile a compendium of medical and treatment information.

This book should be used as a companion to the other resources already available. I have listed these associations in the Resources Section of the book. Foundation staff often hear, with a great sigh of frustration and relief, "Oh, only if I had known you were here a year ago!" There will be many questions and needs that you will have beyond the scope of this book and they are there to help you.

The intent of the book is to cover some common areas of concern; to share with you some personal examples of how others have dealt with their diagnosis and recovery, and to acknowledge the struggle you are going through. The following stories are divided into three sections; patient stories; family stories; and professional caregivers' stories.

Part Two

Chapter Two

Patients Tell How They Cope

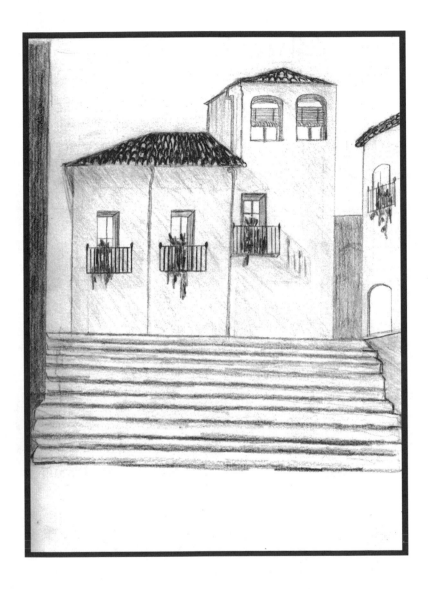

Surround Yourself with Those You Love: Kristan's Story

Kristan Elizabeth Randolf was born in Chicago, Illinois and grew up mostly in Des Moines, Iowa. She currently is single and living in Oakland, CA. Before her illness, she did mental health counseling full-time and therapeutic massage in the evenings. She enjoys swimming, biking, dancing, shopping, going out for lunch, reading, hanging out with her family and friends, and loves animals. In 1993 Kris had surgery for a glioblastoma grade IV. She has had no recurrence of the tumor.

In late 1991, I began to have some problems: frequent headaches that nothing could touch, strange bodily experiences that felt like energy rushing through my body and out the top of my head. By February of 1992, the headaches were so severe that I felt nauseated, and at times was unable to remain upright, saw blotches, and was unable to focus visually.

The first time I went to my regular physician, she said that I was having "tension headaches" and prescribed exercise, but did agree to do some tests to see if there was any "medical cause." I called in March and was told that all of my tests were normal and "you're fine." At the beginning of April, I saw another physician, who referred me to psychiatry and prescribed pain medication. My boyfriend had become increasingly worried, and when I became disoriented, he convinced me to go to the hospital. After having a CAT scan, I was admitted on May 9, with a "large mass" in my brain. Within thirty-six hours, I had gone into a coma and had emergency surgery.

The diagnosis was glioblastoma multiforme, grade four. The tumor was the size of a lemon, located in my right frontal lobe crossing the midline. After surgery (subtotal resection) I was referred to UCSF medical facility and agreed to take part in a study. The treatment was to be aggressive, because this is an aggressive tumor. I had radiation twice daily with DFMO, an oral radiosensitizer, for four and half weeks.

I do not remember the week preceding surgery or the few days following it. What I first remember is my boyfriend sitting next to me, holding an ice pack on my head for eight hours at a time. My mom and stepdad had come from Des Moines, sister from San Diego. I was disoriented and thought that they lived here. They stayed in my apartment, during my two weeks in the hospital, staying to visit me for eight hours every day. My mom brought me fruit salads, because I refused to eat the tofu enchilada that came twice every day. My friends came after work and during work, despite the fact that I had been transferred to Redwood City, which was about forty-five minutes away.

The social worker from the hospital told my family and best friend that I would never be the same; that I would be unable to drive or to live alone. Fortunately, no one relayed the news to me, so I kept getting better.

My mother stayed with me, in my studio apartment for four months following surgery, dropping her own life in Des Moines. She was my prime support, social worker, and good buddy. Did we have fun together, and I couldn't have done it without her.

I read lots of books given to me by my sister, friends, and friends of my family. I practiced visualizing the tumor being swept away or eaten by animals. I expected the tumor to be completely gone by the end of treatment. In August, I was completely shocked, when I learned from my oncologist that this tumor usually reoccurs, and that people die from it. I changed oncologists.

After the initial shock, activity kept me from thinking about the prognosis. My major fear was that others would not be able to go on without me.

My MRI immediately following the treatment was better than any of the doctors expected. The tumor had shrunk amazingly. Two months later it looked even better. I have scans every two months for the first year. After my next one, it will go to every three months. Currently, there has been no growth, and I am in remission. As a part of the protocol at UCSF, I will be monitored by them for ten years, as well as my regular doctors.

Some major factors are impacting my recovery: my positive attitude and that of those around me, laughter, lots of love from so many people, their prayers from all around the world, and good medical treatment. Even on the bad days (like when I lost hair from radiation) Mom and I maintained a sense of humor. I am so thankful to have had the whole summer with my mother.

I had read about people who said that they were thankful for their diseases, dismissing them as crazy. Eight months later, I am one of them. My life has changed dramatically, and I love every day of my life, even the hard ones. I appreciate the richness of my emotions. I feel more passionate about things, about making each day precious. This has brought me closer to my family and friends. I have met other long time survivors, which has be inspirational.

As far as advice to anyone, I would say to surround yourself with those whom you love. Get involved in support groups. Read positive thinkers, like Bernie Siegel. Practice visualization (drawing the picture first helps.) Go easy on yourself; expect to take some time for effects to lessen. Explore alternative treatments as an adjunct to Western medicine. Keep pressing your doctors, when you know something is happening with you. They are not inside of your body. Talk about your fears; other people have them too. Do not let anyone tell you how long you have to live. They can only recite statistics.

A Happy Ending After a Long and Confusing Journey: Laura's Story

Laura was diagnosed at age 25 as having ganglioneuroma, a rare form of tumor which contains cells from the neurons and from tissue in between the nerve cells and blood vessels. It is a slow growing tumor , usually treated with surgery, and occurs in the brain or spinal cord. She has had no recurrence of the tumor since surgery. Laura is single, lives in Daly City, California and works in customer service. In her spare time she enjoys skiing, biking, walking and reading.

It was the summer of 1985 and a very exciting time in my life. I had just graduated from high school, and was looking forward to going to college. After going to Hawaii to celebrate my graduation, I went to Lake Tahoe for the 4th of July. I don't know if the fireworks had any effect on me, but that was when I had my first seizure. I just so happened to be sharing a room with my mom who woke up during the episode. Since I was not prone to having seizures she panicked and thought the worst. She called Emergency and an ambulance arrived. I woke up with paramedics in my room and totally confused. At first I would not agree to go to the hospital but my family convinced me to go. The doctor who was treating me said that I had a grand mal seizure.

When I came home I saw my regular physician. She referred me to a neurologist. The neurologist had me have a CAT scan and EEG test. All of my tests came out normal. After all the 'fun' tests, the neurologist concluded I had epilepsy. He said I may have had other seizures but since I sleep alone no one would have known. He prescribed Dilantin. I filled the prescription but decided to not take the medication. I was not convinced I had epilepsy and did not want to take pills I did not feel I needed.

During that time I had an intercom hooked up in my room to monitor my sleep. My family did not want me to be alone in fear that I would have another seizure. Since I did not see myself have the seizures I had a hard time understanding their concern. Well, nothing happened. To this day I have not experienced another grand mal seizure.

Three years later I started having psychomotor seizures. I would feel nervous, turn red in the face, get a metal like taste in my mouth and feel queasy in the stomach. The symptoms were so mild that only I knew I was having the spell. They lasted for a few months. Since the term "psychomotor seizures" had not been introduced to me I called the seizure spells. I went back to the same neurologist who still felt I had epilepsy. However, I was still not sold on the diagnosis and felt the spells were stress related. The first seizure happened after a stressful time in my life and these seizures started occurring when I was preparing to graduate from junior college and changing jobs. I thought the spells may have been a fright/flight response.

Two years later "they were back." As in the past, I was going through a stressful time in my life. I was getting ready to graduate from college and begin my career. The seizure I had two years ago were mild in comparison to these. They happened more frequently, from once to twice a week, to every day. At times they occurred more than once a day. Being stressed or worried seemed to provoke them. With time the episodes seemed to last longer. Ranging from a few seconds to a minute. Half of the time no one would know I was having a spell. At times I wasn't sure if in fact I had one and at other times I would tell whoever I was with that I was having one. They would pass and then I would be back to whatever I was doing.

The more frequently the seizures happened the more I became concerned. These spells were not going away as the others had in the past. Reluctantly I went back to the neurologist. I described the spells and he called them psychomotor seizures. That was the first time I had heard that term. I still called them spells because I hated the "S" word. I was schedule to have an MRI. The result showed a slow growing glioma. Of course all possibilities had to be ruled out, such as if I had been in a foreign country where I could have eaten raw meat and caught a parasite which showed up as scar tissue on the scan.

Navigating Through a Strange Land

My neurologist said the words glioma, temporal lobe, and cyst. I was so confused. At the time I was seeing an endocrinologist who recommended that I see a neurosurgeon. The neurosurgeon used all the same words my neurologist used. I just wanted to know what the difference between cyst, glioma, and tumor was. According to the neurosurgeon I was better off having the tumor alone. It was slow growing and had not changed size: It was best to just monitor it . Well those words were all I heard and thought I was off the hook.

My endocrinologist called me later that week to discuss my appointment with the neurosurgeon. He went through the doctors notes and for the first time I heard the diagnosis clearly. I had a ganglioneuroma in the right side of my temporal lobe. He encouraged me to get a second opinion.

The second doctor confirmed the diagnosis and said I should have had the tumor removed a long time ago. He was so cut and dry about the whole thing. I just sat in my chair and felt as though my stomach fell to the floor. I was speechless. From hearing one doctor saying to leave it alone to hearing I should have brain surgery was something I did not expect. I thought he would have agreed with the original diagnosis. I was in shock. I could not even comprehend the idea of brain surgery. It sounded so barbaric. I was dead set against it. There was no way I was going to have my head cut open. I made up my mind to not have the surgery. There was just no way I was going to risk my life.

Patients Tell How They Cope

A few days later I opened the newspaper and there was a full blown article on the doctor I had seen for the second opinion. At first I threw the paper aside but later read the article. I decided to follow his advice and get a third opinion before I made up my mind. Before going to the appointment I went to a health library and spent hours reading about brain surgery, alternative medicine and defining all of the medical terms that were being thrown at me. Also I called the Brain Tumor Foundation to get informational booklets such as The Guide, sent to me. I became obsessed in learning all I could.

The third neurosurgeon agreed with the second. He said it would be best to take the tumor out as well as the epileptic seizures. At that moment I knew that surgery was the right thing to do. Without a doubt, I said let's do it. My mom just looked at me as if she were hearing things. She was with me when I saw the second doctor and knew how I had felt about surgery prior to that moment. That day I made the arrangements.

On February 18, 1992 I had my surgery at a Kaiser Hospital. I came out of surgery with flying colors. Before the actual surgery I really prepared myself mentally, physically and spiritually. I had a positive attitude toward surgery and knew I would be fine. I visualized coming out of surgery and the doctor telling me the tumor was totally removed. Above all I would not have seizures. I would be normal again. Also my MRI would be clear. I also attended brain tumor support group meetings. It was such a help meeting others who had gone through surgery and lived. It was also reassuring to know I was not the only one in the world with a tumor. I asked the nurses and members as many questions as I could.

The surgery was a success. I had no permanent side effects. However, I developed aseptic meningitis from the surgery. The surgery was nothing compared to the meningitis. I woke up with the worst headache after surgery. I was prepared for some pain but this was beyond words. Some members in the support group said I would have no pain, but not me. There was no magic pill to cure the meningitis. I just had to wait for the blood in my spinal fluid to work its way out. So for two months I had daily headaches and back pain.

One of my biggest fears was waking up after surgery and looking like a beast. At least I did not have to loose all of my hair and only the section where the tumor was located. I was so concerned with my hair that I even asked my surgeon to diagram the area he had to remove so I could plan an alternate hairstyle with my stylist. Luckily I have thick curly hair because I was able to part my hair on the opposite side and cover the area where I had my surgery.

Initially after surgery I had trouble with short term memory, as well as thinking of the right words I wanted to use in the present moment. At first I was frustrated but I worked with my memory by associating something with what I wanted to remember. In time my memory improved. In fact people around me could see a difference. I also experienced "circuit overload." This is what other people in the support group characterized as what happened to them when there was just too much going on around them at once. At first it was new to me but I learned to work with it. I still experience the circuit overload as well as not being able to recall the right word for what I want to say.

Follow up care consisted of annual six month MRI scanning. Later this year I will have a scan every year. After surgery I was taking Dilantin. Since I did not have a seizure after surgery my neurologist and neurosurgeon decided I could get off of the medication completely.

At first the idea of brain surgery was out of the question for me. Then I did my research. I felt that this was my head and my body. I recommend anyone in the same situation to become involved in their illness. The doctor's throw so much at you at once that unless you take control you will feel powerless. The Brain Tumor Foundation provides the patient and their family with a wealth of information.

At first I couldn't stand to see the brain tumor letterhead on the envelopes in my mail. But once I accepted the fact of my condition those guides and pamphlets were such helpful resources. Becoming involved in a support group is another strong recommendation I give to anyone facing any health crisis. I attended a meeting two weeks before surgery and three weeks after my surgery.

Navigating Through a Strange Land

The members of the group that had the surgery were so inspirational to me before I had my surgery that I went back afterward. I was an inspiration to new people at the meeting. Since my surgery went so well I was able to give others hope.

It took seven years to finally diagnose my condition. After going through such an ordeal I realized that not only did I have the tumor but everyone I know and didn't know had the tumor as well. It affected everyone I knew and those that were close to them. Because I am a private person I didn't tell anyone I knew about my condition. I kept it to myself and my immediate family. It wasn't until the day before I went to get a third opinion that I told my co-workers. From there I told my friends and others family members. Once I got started I couldn't keep quiet. It felt so good to talk about my problem with people that were close to me.

Since my surgery I have become more open and do not hold all of my feelings inside. After I told people, I was overwhelmed by the support I received. The love and support from my family and friends had to be the best medicine during my recovery.

Asking questions is another important tool to getting through the surgery. Every morning I would have a notebook ready with a list of things I wanted to go over with my doctor. I also had the phone numbers of people in my support group to fall back on as well as volunteers from the National Brain Tumor Foundation.

Patients Tell How They Cope

When you live through a crisis like this other problems seem so trivial. A cold is nothing and the flu is a piece of cake. After surgery I appreciated life so much more and reevaluated my personal direction. I went through a whole period of being totally unsatisfied with everything including my job and house.

It was a very difficult time. I felt as though I was satisfied with my life before surgery but totally unsatisfied with everything after. I felt that I was given a second chance and didn't want to waste a second of my life. In time, I came to grips with these feelings and made positive changes and as a result of them I learned a lot about myself.

When you are pushed against a wall you definitely become a stronger and more worldly person with a deeper connection to the universe. If anything, you appreciate the simple things in life, like waking up in the morning and being able to open your eyes, see the sky, get out of bed and put your feet on the ground.

Healing Is a Lifelong Process:

Marie's Story

Marie was born in Salt Lake City, Utah and raised in Southern California. She has lived in San Francisco for the past 23 years with her husband and son. Marie works at a coffee house part-time, and enjoys quilting, and reading mysteries in her spare time. Marie was diagnosed with a meningioma on her fifth cranial nerve. She subsequently had two operations and radiation therapy. Currently, the tumor is gone, but there are some minor aftereffects.

The odyssey began a lifetime ago, or so it seems to me now. Most of it is kind of a blur, but it is easiest for me to remember the sequence of events as they relate to milestones in our son's life. His name is Aaron and he will be eleven on July 2, 1993. Together with my husband Larry, we live in the Sunset district in San Francisco.

In February of 1988, Aaron was in his second semester of kindergarten. A small meningioma was discovered, quite by accident. It was attached to the fifth cranial nerve, the one to the right side of my face. But I was completely asymptomatic. What the doctor was searching for was the cause of the severe vertigo I had been experiencing for the past year. The first two attacks were so debilitating that I was bedridden for a week each time, unable to even lift my head from the pillow. The third attack left me with ringing in the ears, loss of hearing in one ear, and a loss of balance for months.

After seeing several neurosurgeons, it was determined that the meningioma had nothing to do with the vertigo. The meningioma was monitored regularly, and I began a series of tests for the vertigo.

In May of 1989, Aaron was completing the first grade. I began to have tingling sensations on the right side of my face, just under the eye. They were intermittent and painless. By the time Aaron began the second grade, in September of 1989, the meningioma had shown some signs of growth. I had surgery a week after school began. The neurosurgeon was able to remove most, but not all, of the tumor, because of its location. Recovery went well and I was back to work in two months.

In May of 1990, the pain began. It was at first very quick, like a flash of light, in the area of my teeth, both top and bottom on the right side. I didn't know what it was, it all happened so fast. The next occurrence was about two months later. This time, the pain lasted a minute or two longer. Gradually, these attacks became closer together, lasting longer each time, until November, when the pain became continuous. It was a searing, electrical pain that sometimes caused the right side of my face to vibrate from the intensity. It didn't seem to matter what activity or non-activity I was engaged in. It would even wake me from a deep sleep. Talking and eating became extremely difficult. I was no longer able to read to Aaron, so he read to me.

In the meantime, I discovered a small lump in my right breast. It was removed in October, 1990. The pathologist found that it contained abnormal cells, but decided it was benign. It is monitored regularly.

My neurosurgeon felt that radiation therapy was in order for the meningioma. After getting a second opinion at UC Medical Center, I began my treatment in mid-November, 1990. They were administered five days a week, for six weeks.

During this time, I experienced a great deal of fatigue and nausea. It reminded me of the first trimester of pregnancy. The radiation also affected my sense of taste; everything I ate tasted like soap. I began to have trouble keeping food down, my weight began to drop, and my head and face felt hot and dry to the touch. One day, as I left radiation therapy, it began to rain lightly. I have a vivid memory of how cool and refreshing the raindrops felt as they touched my face.

Midway through the treatments, the pain became excruciating from the swelling of the tumor. The dexamethasone helped immensely with the pain and the loss of appetite. I was soon eating everything in sight. I quickly gained back the lost pounds and then some. I suddenly had an enormous amount of energy. I began cleaning things I'd never cleaned before or at least not for a very long time. I cooked things I had never cooked before. And through all of this, I slept only about three hours a night.

I completed the treatments just after New Year's, 1991. There was some hair loss above both ears, and just above the forehead. This was a temporary condition, and the new growth began to come in within the month. The facial pain, however, continued to plague me. I began taking Tegretol, in February of 1991. At first, I took a very small dose, just half a tablet a day. I did not feel any pain, or anything else for that matter. I didn't even feel the floor I was waking on. I was floating. But this "floaty" feeling disappeared after a while, and very soon, I was taking much larger doses.

By the following year, it was clearly not working for me any longer. The pain seemed to be unaffected by the drug, and the side effects became unbearable. I began to have double "rolling" vision. It was like watching a television set whose vertical hold control no longer worked, causing the picture to keep moving upwards. The two images that I saw were stacked, one on top of the other. It made me feel nauseous.

Because I could no longer control the pain through the use of drugs, I went back into surgery. This time my doctor was performing a rhizotomy to sever the fifth cranial nerve, but cutting only the part that corresponded to the area of pain in my face. I was looking forward to this operation, thinking that I would finally be pain-free. But to my disappointment, when I regained consciousness in the recovery room, the pain was still there. I also had some rather strange symptoms.

In the hospital, I developed an itch on the right side of my forehead. Whenever I would scratch it, I would feel the scratching on the top of my head. I still feel that itchy feeling every now and then, but I never again experienced the scratching sensation on the top of my head whenever I scratched my forehead. But no matter how much I scratch my forehead, the itch is never satisfied. I also had a numbing sensation on my right eyelid, the right side of my nose, and the right side of my upper lip.

The good news was that my doctor was able to see that the tumor was completely gone. Only scar tissue remained. The radiation had done its job. The MRI's since the first craniotomy had always indicated that the tumor was still there, even after radiation. But apparently the scar tissue was what was showing up. I was greatly relieved to know the tumor was gone.

At the present time, almost a year since the rhizotomy, the level of pain is quite low, and I am not taking any medication for the pain. It was a very gradual process getting to this point. I have had a strange taste in my mouth (slightly salty, slightly sour) constantly since the rhizotomy. Intermittently, I get a sensation on the right side of my forehead that feels like an insect is crawling down my forehead from the hairline to the eyebrow and then back up again. I once experienced a period of about two weeks of intense activity under my right eye, twitching and spasms day and night, followed by about six weeks of painlessness.

The journey has been a long one. And I'm sure it isn't over yet, but somehow I feel the worst is past. I have come to realize that healing is a lifelong process. In this process the support group has played a major role, as well as my husband and son. Having Larry and Aaron provided me with enormous motivation for getting well and made difficult decisions somehow seem clear-cut. In many ways, my life has become better. By prioritizing and eliminating the less important things, I have improved the quality of my life. And so, I live my life one day at a time, taking nothing for granted.

Navigating Through a Strange Land

A 20-Year Survivor of a
Craniopharyngioma: Kris's Story

Kris was diagnosed with a craniopharyngioma at age 16, after many years of being treated for an underactive thyroid. These tumor/cysts occur around the optic nerves and hypothalamus, near the pituitary gland. It is formed from left over cells from fetal development. Just ten years ago it was considered inoperable. Kris did have surgery, 20 years ago, by the then-experimental transphenoidal surgery, but the pituitary gland had to be removed. She has been on replacement hormones since then. Today the transphenoidal (or through the nasal passage) is the standard procedure used for most pituitary tumors, and is usually very effective in all but the most insidious tumors. Kris was a speaker at the 1992 National Brain Tumor Foundation conference. A native Oregonian, she lives outside of Portland, Oregon and enjoys exploring ocean beaches; nature hikes; travel; creating; gardening; massage and reading.

My childhood was plagued with the normal childhood illnesses, plus a few more earaches and skin rashes than most. Around second grade, my parents became concerned with my height for which they sought answers from our family pediatrician. By fourth grade, I had stopped growing altogether. By my early teens, no sign of puberty had blossomed and my three year younger sister was sprouting past me. Naps helped me recharge for I felt drained dealing with the pace, demands, and peer-group pressures of school. I frequently carried around a glass of ice-water to satisfy my craving thirst. I never slept soundly in a consistent pattern. As I aged, the illness or accidents seem to be more than my sibling. I broke both of my legs skiing, and I missed a term of school due to pneumonia.

For about nine years, the pediatrician monitored my condition through blood test chemistries, and height and weight measurements. Synthyroid was prescribed during all this time, for what was diagnosed as an under-functioning thyroid. My normal growth did not improve during this regimen.

Going to the doctor regularly for tests was a routine I thought everyone did. But slowly I realized this wasn't so. I started learning and feeling my differences.

When I was in tenth grade, my mother read a magazine article about growth hormone, which provided the clue to discovering the true cause of my stunted growth. Mom called the doctor at home late that evening discussing the symptoms and findings in this article. Within a short time, an appointment was scheduled to x-ray my head to address my mom's concerns.

I still remember hearing the sentence as clearly today as it was 20 years ago. Walking towards the patient exam room, I met my doctor mid-hall as he was scurrying from one room to the next. He announced his findings in the hall, within earshot of any passersby and the open doors of patients rooms. We stood standing face-to- face as he announced with a look of seriousness in his eyes, "there's a dark mass that is abnormal in your brain, could be a brain tumor, but I'm not sure what it is."

My doctor was a jolly sort who frequently used humor, candy, a lovable disposition, and warm hugs in his practice. I thought he was kidding, since I had become accustomed to his jokes. He said he was not joking, ushered me to my exam room, and asked me to wait, that he'd be there in just a moment. In those moments, I experienced a wave of feelings more intense than any other I could remember. My shock turned to terror with a churning mix of anxiety, and confusion in my stomach. How could this be true? Maybe he has the wrong patient. Certainly this couldn't be me he was talking about. He entered the room and offered me the customary Dummy-brand lollipop.

I was a minor (16 years old) and my parents were not with me. Trips to the doctor's office were frequent and a part of my routine where I would go after school for a blood test. A family member would meet me or pick-me up after work. He showed me the x-rays, and referred me to a neurosurgery group for a more conclusive diagnosis, and treatment options. In 1974, these x-rays simply showed a dark abnormal indeterminable mass. I still can see those x-rays in my mind. I left the office feeling like I had been hit with a steamroller, shocked, scared, smashed. I met my mom in the parking lot, sharing my experience and the manner the doctor presented all this to me. She went in to talk with him.

The appointment to speak with the neurosurgeon seemed like a very long wait. The waiting and not knowing made me dwell on my worst fears. Would I survive, and if I survived would I be normal , or a coma vegetable like my mom's friend who had a tumor. Finally we met with the neurosurgeon; he handled our discussion with gentleness and concern.

Many long and painful tests ensued for about another month. Every part of my body felt not-private, probed, explored and viewed. I was quickly learning to disassociate myself; feeling instead like a guinea pig and embarrassed to be so exposed. I hurt everywhere. My hands and arms were so bruised and crippled from all the needles. I had to have a very painful IV stuck in my hands and arms to feed medications and to take the tests, since my veins were little and unproductive after all the needles. I couldn't even handle my own silverware to eat my favorite food (watermelon). The hospital nurses were like friends. They seemed to understand why I cried when it felt so great to bath in a tub after many long tests. Back rubs, smiles and doing the hospital recreation art projects all helped during this time.

I was frequently moved in with the victim of a drunk

driving car wreck. The tracheotomy and tubes and her listlessness still haunt me. The noise from all the medical contraptions around her were grotesque. Not a very positive experience before possibly going into surgery myself.

The pre-operative test results were inconclusive and surgery was recommended to further determine what exactly the gray-mass was. Surgery was scheduled for July 3, 1974. From the first doctor's x-rays to the surgery last about 3 months.

Every station seemed to have something medical on it. The night before my surgery, the show I watched was about a brain tumor patient who died. A psychologist came to speak to me. I still don't know who requested him, but it wasn't my request. We discussed my preferences of hot & cold. I vaguely remember a conversation about a comment I made about death. The psychologist's gaze grew more stern and we spent more moments than most discussing his concern with my thoughts. I also was visited by the hospital priest and our church's priest.

Flowers, gifts, and cards with lots of visits from family and friends helped. But, seeing many people I did not see very often made me alarmed. A feeling of doom seemed to pass in their handshakes, kisses, & hugs of support. Something was wrong despite well-meaning assurances. I could feel it.

Finally, the day of reckoning came. The nurse harpooned my rear with painkillers. Dad's reassuring hand clasp and tearful desire to exchange places with me if possible; mom's ghost-blanched face were final thoughts as hospital staff wheeled me down the long hallway toward the elevators that would carry me to the operating room. The last friend I saw was my Godmother, mid hall with flowers and gifts, as I was being rolled away.

I remember feeling like I might die; but did not tell my parents about my fears because I was afraid of adding a burden to their already troubled faces. I think people's reactions, the psychologist, priests, the television show, memories of my mom's tumor friend in a nursing home, and seeing a lot of people I did not normally see all added to this feeling that I wasn't going to make it. Who knows how to talk to a child in a way a kid can understand. Direct and simple is helpful. Acting like everything will be ok does not make things better when your feelings tell you otherwise.

The anesthesiologist dripped something in an IV that ached into my swollen, bruised hands and wrist. I remember asking him some questions about hurting and staring at the pod-like round bright surgical lights. Painting surgical rooms' ceilings with pleasant nature scenes may be a good idea, was my final thought as I drifted off to sleep.

I awoke to the conscious world with a cousin I infrequently saw, perched at my table side, next to a row of fellow surgical recoverees. There was an unrelenting clanging from the jingle-bells tied to the patient's toes next to me, and a walloping feeling of head and body pain. I had to remain absolutely still and lay flat. No cushy pillows, just a hard bed and a few cool blankets. There was a thunder & lightening storm with heavy rains. I could really hear and feel this. Noise and light were such irritants!

After the $5^1/_2$ hour surgery, I mentally checklisted my wholeness. I had experienced a complication of some spinal fluid leakage and blood loss. I couldn't feel the sensation of my hands on my upper right leg. No one told me why until later. I thought I had lost part of my leg. A muscle graft was used to patch the cavity where the pituitary and tangerine-sized cyst once were. My nose was packed with sponge-like gauze from the new transphenoidal surgical procedure (an incision going between the inside upper lip and front teeth, then through the nasal passage to the pituitary cavity). I had tape, stitches, tubes, and discoloring antiseptics everywhere. I concentrated on a teakettle sound to relieve the throbbing everywhere I seemed to bring my consciousness.

I was kept in a private, dark, and quiet room (per my request), with only the small blinking red light of a room monitor in the upper left corner of the room. I remember having a lot of bad nightmares, waking to a shaking feeling of the bed (or was it me), and no one to reach out for. My family was with me most of the time, but had to change watch for sleep and work. This ordeal was long and hard on my whole family.

Within a short time, walking was encouraged. I was afraid to do this for the point to "lay flat and still" was drilled into me. Within 10 days of brain surgery, I meandered through a neighborhood summer festival. I drove to the ocean with my mom. This was the first place I wanted to go after surgery. The ocean still replenishes me today just like it did then.

They removed the cyst, but they also removed the pituitary gland. At the time they thought this growth was from the pituitary and so took out the entire thing. It was determined that hormonal therapy and routine medical monitoring would be needed for the rest of my life. These drugs helped to manage unquenchable thirst for cold water, moderate frequent urination, and correct interrupted sleep habits, balance mood swings and boost energy.

However, part of me died during all these procedures and with the operation. A new way to experience life emerged. I quit "living" life, feeling, and trusting. I felt alienated from my peer group, family, friends, and physicians. I quit allowing myself to feel grief, joy, or whatever. I became very much a doer, a task oriented person.

I was angry and trying to deny this had happened to me. It was interfering with dating, high school activities, and dreams that now seemed shattered. I was dealing with a personality that was alien to me. My body did things that was uncomfortable. There were many things I could no longer do, like swimming which I loved.

Navigating Through a Strange Land

After surgery, I gained a tremendous amount of weight. I couldn't understand all these strange changes in my body and mind. It didn't seem like my body anymore. There didn't seem to be anyone I felt safe enough to talk to without possibly experiencing ridicule. I remember vividly, right after surgery, being in the grocery store at the checkout line. A little girl pulled her mom's skirt and said, "Look mommy, it's Frankenstein." My legs had iodine and stitches and scars on them from the graft. Comments like these really hurt me.

I think that people were there trying to reach-out to me but I had shut them out in my mind and feelings and couldn't see it that way then. All I remember hearing, especially as I got older, was "you're so lucky, isn't that enough? or "can't you just get on with life and quit thinking about it so much." These comments seem to be subtle put-downs and reminders I was not okay in the eyes of others, since these comments came at the times I tried to express my feelings.

For the next fifteen years I was regularly monitored to make sure the hormone therapies were in balance, to lead a normal life-style.

In 1989, after consistent daily medication, I elected to abstain from all supplements to see how my body would react autonomously. I craved and strongly felt that there was something better than the way I was living. I thought, "I have just this one chance at this life, and I will do my best to have it be my best." I felt I needed a different approach to my condition.

However, instead of improving my condition, it set me back for about 2 years. My request to go off all medications started me on a whirlwind of suicidal and depressive thoughts. I had barely enough energy just to go make a living and return home. Exhausted, I'd collapse in bed. I felt like I was losing the one thing I had always been able to count on... my mind. I would hear strange sounds and experience alarming shudders at night. I did not like being around people, noise or questions. I became reclusive.

I did a lot of intensive soul-searching because I thought it was 'me' who was depressed. I found out much later that this suicidal-like depression was a reaction from going off some of the medication.

In 1991, I changed physicians because my long-term endocrinologist was near retirement. I found a new endocrinologist, retested for abnormal brain growths, changed some brands of medication, as well as added a few new ones. These changes proved to be very fruitful. I was elated to go through puberty finally! I was thirty-three years old when I developed into a more womanly body. I no longer felt fears of being rejected for my child-like body. I quit beating myself up for something I couldn't change. I was told I could possibly bear children!

A strong communicative relationship with my new endocrinologist allowed fine-tuning of my quest to feel health, happiness, and joy to the best of my ability every day. Knowing what makes me tick and keeping a record of the subtle nuances of my body helped piece the puzzle together.

I have a personal physician who I believe understands how to live well himself. Empathy (not sympathy), and an interest to see something in a new way, was important for an objective and helpful approach to an old struggle. Feelings and actions override any words.

As a child, I felt many times I was not given the time to discuss my concerns and observations. Just enough time was allowed to answer the standard routine questions of what prescriptions, have this test, and briefly discuss the results in medical jargon I did not understand. As an adult, I have learned to find physicians that I can express myself with. I have also learned to be more honest about my feelings with my doctor.

In 1992, I was a guest speaker at the second annual National Brain Tumor Convention. My college friend, Tricia Roloff, who was diagnosed with a brain tumor several years after college, talked me into going to this conference. It was my first experience of going public with 'my secret.' I am so appreciative to have met so many survivors of brain tumors. Sharing has opened many wonderful doorways and lessened the fear of coping. Truly, this one single event has powerfully influenced me to have the courage to live the way I want to live.

I began listening and sharing more in many aspects of my life. My relationships improved in all areas. My friend asked me to join her in an art therapy class. I loved creating without any performance evaluation! I studied and experienced many alternative health and wellness techniques. I tried things many people had not heard about like light and color therapy.

I studied life-style simplifying, environments, electrical energy, chemical ingredients, laws of life, nutrition, relaxation, stretching, breathing. I surrounded myself with hobbies and people that made me feel good. I became an avid architect of my life-style. I learned to accept my different moods and use them to clarify issues that were bothering me. Instead of pushing a bad feeling away, I listened to what it was trying to tell me. I learned facing your own fears is the first step to true fulfilling happiness and peace.

I decided to give up a stressful job that was negatively effecting my health. For many years I tried to live up to everyone else's expectations of how I should be living my life; to be like everyone else. I worked very hard, achieving many awards in my field. But, the monetary compensation from my demanding job no longer outweighed the damage it was doing to me, physically and psychologically. I wanted a peaceful, balanced and healthy life.

My company offered me a leave when I tried to quit. Counseling was offered and encouraged through my employer. For the first time in my life I went to a counselor. My company offered me 2000 hours as a benefit of employment. I was scared their knowledge of the darker side of my health condition would prevent me from having 'normal' opportunities down the road, even though my track record proved me as a consistent hard-working producer. I had seen what had happened to other employees.

I was able to work long enough to sell my home, take care of my medical expenses and get cash for everything I had. I was emotionally wiped out from all the changes in the past several years, including the medication, family deaths and several changes of address. I wanted a chance to fully recuperate with no real responsibilities. Taxes and health insurance costs took a lot of this money, but I had enough to live on for about a year.

The American dream was no longer my idea of dream living. For a year and a half I lived my dream. I experimented with many different life-styles, hobbies, and travels. I camped and slept in nature's quietness. Of course, I lived at the ocean for a while, too. I spoke with other brain tumor survivors, family and other types of patients who had learned to take-back control of their life.

I wrote, read, gardened, explored, hiked, rode horses, and fell in-love for the first time to a man I met while traveling. My fiancé and my relationship made me aware of things I never noticed before. Like, I get moody or pick fights when I take a specific hormone to trigger menses. I had lived single for well over 13 years. Friends and family offered me places to live to recuperate and store the things I kept, and helped brainstorm new careers. They listened and laughed and cried with me.

It's now Spring of 1994 and I now am just trying to rebuild and reenter mainstream again. I still find the old frustrating struggles there to greet me... the peril of trying to take care of the necessities of life by earning a living, balancing daily living, and qualifying for a right to adequate health coverage. I am stronger this time though—rested, healthy. I know the keys to living well for me are positive people and environments, living simply, proper rotated-nutritional diets, a focus on wellness, exercise, rest, sleep, quiet time in nature and doing something I love every day. I used to work in a stress filled environment that adversely affected my wellness and state-of-mind for financial and health benefits security. But, there is no security when their is no health.

I am attempting to combine my hobbies and interests with all my business, sales, marketing, advertising skills to make a living. My first priority is to feel health, peace, and joy every day. My second is to have time to love my fiancé, family and friends. My last priority is to work hard for the sake of money, things, and awards.

I am struggling with trying to obtain my last option for health insurance now that my COBRA benefits are about to expire. After two years of applications, I am awaiting words for acceptance from the Oregon High Risk Health Pool, since my rare condition is virtually uninsurable. This is based on the history of the average of most people with a condition like mine, and not by the merits of my long healthy life.

What has living as a long-term survivor been like? Frustrating, scary, and at times seemingly insurmountably tough. My life-style completely changed as I knew it to be 20 years ago. And it keeps changing. The daily medication and regular doctor visits are vivid reminders of my difference and trauma from my painful and emotionally haunting rollercoaster history. Fear still sneaks back to haunt me at times, and I do get moody, frustrated, and depressed. I am learning the importance of pace and patience, for I still push too hard trying to do it all today. There's some good from all this too. I have developed more of an acceptance of myself and others. I learned I treated other people with more consideration than I gave myself. I learned everyone has something that seems just as traumatic for them and that maybe I'm not so "different."

At times, I seem disassociated from that little girl... that couldn't possibly have happened to me. Yet, my feelings and experiences are etched in my face and body showing the scars and triumphs I have endured. Medical technology, tests, understanding seem so far advanced to the routine medical treatment and tests I experienced growing-up. "Now" seems to offer so many more possibilities for quicker, more accurate, less painful test, and a shorter waiting period for information, relieving the churning anxiety that the fear of not knowing brings. I have witnessed great advances in medical care and understanding. I have also experienced many fears, doubts, and frustrations.

I have worked hard to understand myself. Counseling was not a generally accepted coping strategy then. My mom had always wanted me to feel like I had a normal life and has done everything in her power to help me believe in myself, and to encourage and listen to me when I have had grave doubts and depression. However, emotionally and psychologically pretending to be 'normal' when I felt and saw vast differences that I wasn't the norm, and being forced to comply with 'normally-accepted' ways of acting, thinking, caused me to be ashamed for who I was; embarrassed; and hyper-self-critical (a perfectionist).

I learned that when you look "normal" on the outside, people assume the "inside" is fine too. That hurts. It's like you have to have some defacing abnormality to be justified in your feelings. I felt this frustration not only with my friends, family, but also with the physicians. I hid my feelings, learned how not to feel, and wore a mask of happiness and positive attitude. Mom knows too well the darker side: I swung to suicidal lows and listless depression where I had no energy or worthy reason to get up and make this day happen.

Trying not to focus on all the medical 'treatment' became a big impetus in my life. I began to 'visualize," "dream," and "do" as a diversion, to try to make something in my life more significant than medical issues. The crevice in the bend of my elbows and lower back still cringe when touched a certain way from all the needles and blood tests and pre-operative spinal tap. I learned to listen and be very aware of myself. I also learned there's always at least two ways to look at things. I learned to look without feeling. This in the end, of course, proved harmful.

There's such a fine line between having it all and having nothing… health is the key. It's not enough to be alive and not feel good. I had to learn to face myself by going through a long, painful self-analysis to see what made me tick and react. Books and research became my best friends for companionship and understanding to squelch my fears. I had to really accept myself, to learn to feel OK about things I didn't particularly like about myself. Sharing and allowing others to see me vulnerable is something I just started doing within the last five years again. A good 15 years after surgery.

I encourage physicians to be very sensitive to the tone and feeling you convey in your behavior and be careful not to use humor to deny or lighten what may be a traumatic patient experience. Knowledge without grace can delay/kill the wisdom and faith of the patients body to heal. Make time in your practice where both patient and doctor respect and learn from each other, not in theory but in actual practice. Actually, friends and family too could benefit a patient in this way. Families can research about a condition in a library. Asking, challenging and denying your child/parent of his experience does not help them cope. Make it OK to discuss the good with the bad.

Deep true friendships and a strong drive to taste life were the glue that held me together. My friends help me sort my rational/irrational feelings and the necessary from the desperate. They cared and loved me just as I was with no pretenses. I think they were the ones that helped me learn how to accept myself more. When my college friend had surgery, that was a start —someone to talk to. She became a major link to help me bond, feel trust, and closeness with people again. All my actions in the past several years—changing jobs, trying out new things to help me live a more balanced life— were underlined by these key friends who believed and supported me. Without their love, devotion, acceptance, understanding, care and friendship, I might not be here today.

Who would have thought I would feel so successful in all this loss. Truly this seeming curse has become a blessing. I thank God for my life; my self for faith; and doctors, friends, and family for never giving-up on me even at moments when I did. I have found that I am enjoying life more now that I feel, cry, and do more of what I want to every day. I feel like I have more control, less fear, more choices, and better coping tools.

Navigating Through a Strange Land

One of the most profound things I've learned in all these years is: when you feel a desire, go with it. When I acted against these hunches, the pulse of life's direction became difficult. Learn to listen, appreciate, respect, and trust your intuition. When I didn't, my soul dried-up and my body became weary, exhausted and burned-out. That intuition's intelligent voice keeps my options open, a sense of freedom/choice, and feeling of security in my day.

In all, I believe it is every person's responsibility for his/her own health, despite employers, politicians, government's, and the insurance companies' mirage that they will take care of you. No one can understand you better than yourself.

I have shared with you my story as a 20 year survivor to give you hope, care and encouragement to be truthful with yourself and to do the things that will help you best. You have something special to contribute in this world. Make sure you give yourself an environment that encourages health and healing so that you can feel your best every day.

I Could Now Do All the Things I Dreamed About: Norman's Story

Norman wrote this story for Search in 1988, and is reprinted with his permission. He lives in Walnut Creek, California with his wife and children. After his original diagnosis in 1982, he was told that he had a 20% chance of living another two years. He has had five surgeries (two seed implants, and two to remove necrosis, but has had no recurrence of the tumor) radiation and chemotherapy. Despite his prognosis, he is alive and well. After this article he contributed an article entitled "Handicap provisions: a review and assessment," for the magazine Building Standards; May/June issue, 1990. It traces the history of the Americans with Disabilities Act, and the unified building codes for the disabled. Norman was in the building profession before going on disability after surgery.

This had to be the most difficult decision of my life. I had decided that I was no longer capable of continuing my job. The cancer and associated treatment had won the battle; but I was determined it was not going to win the war. Turning around an old saying, "the body was willing but the mind was weak." Actually, both my mind and body were weak.

Navigating Through a Strange Land

There were so many questions. First was the matter of finances. How would I be able to support myself, my wife, and two small children? After all, I was pulling in a damn good income. Luckily, my employer had a good disability insurance plan. That and social security would get us by. My wife's income from her part-time job would afford us a little more discretionary income. What I did not foresee is how the system entraps you. If my wife made more than $510 a month, we would receive less social security. Any dollar I would make would be deducted from the insurance benefit, social security, or both. Here I was, thirty-nine years old, and essentially retired.

I had to figure out what I would do with all my time. I would no longer have the opportunity to spend up to sixty hours a week working at a job. I had to reorder my life. It would kill me to become a couch potato, wasting my mind (what was left of it), and my body watching what Newton Minow graciously called the "vast wasteland." What did I want to do? I could now do all those things I dreamed about, but never had time for.

Putting down my priorities was my first step. There were the kids. I would spend more time with them, quality time. I could help them with their studies and homework. We could go places and do things, as long as my left side was not too greatly involved, and I did not have to run or walk too far. What it really became is being chauffeur, tutor, and referee. I could help my wife doing light housework, some of the marketing, and other errands. What I had to realize was that they had lives that did not always include me and they wanted me to be there to help where I could, but give them the room they needed, especially the kids.

That still left the basic question. What should I do with all this free time? I had bought a computer the year before, but had not had much time to work on it. I had always wanted to reorganize our personal financial records. What better way than computerization? With respect to computers, I was a real neophyte. It had been almost twenty years since my college courses, and that's generations in terms of computers. I decided that the best way to learn is to do, so I wrote my own programs. It was fun when I finally got them to work, although it was frustrating along the way.

Once that was in place, I only had to do maintenance on the programs. What would I do next? I had heard that there is a great story in everybody. I had also heard that if you are to write, write about something you know. I always wanted to write a book. I had written a number of articles for technical periodicals, but that is a very different style of writing. I decide to write the first of what I hoped would become a number of books, using a character much like myself.

It has been a year since I started. That book is now in a semifinal draft, and I am well into my second effort, a mystery. I do not know if my book is publishable, but that is almost irrelevant; I did it, and I am pleased with my accomplishment. The nice thing about writing for me is I am under no pressure, no deadlines, other than my own, and if I don't feel like writing one day, I don't have to. If I am motivated I can sit at the computer all day. I can work an hour, two hours, or not at all. This freedom is something I don't remember ever having before. It is the single most recognizable benefit of my disability; I have the freedom to set my own schedule with very few restrictions.

Ever since my diagnosis in 1982, I have accepted one fact: life is a series of adjustments. Sometimes these adjustments are forced upon us, such as the adjustments to the effects of a chronic disease. Rarely do we get a chance to decide what adjustments we want to make. The realization that my chosen career and my days of being intimately involved in that world were over, made me take a few short steps backward to assess what the rest of my life could and should be. The choices I made were what was right for me, not necessarily the next guy.

There is one thing that should never change in anyone; we have to accept things as they are, but cherish the most wonderful gift that we ever get, life. It is up to each and every person to make their own decisions as how to best use that gift in the best way they can for whatever purposes they believe are the most important to themselves. It is then up to the individual to go do it.

Experimenting with RU 486:

Fume's Story

Fume is single, does general office work, and in her spare time likes reading and sports. She was diagnosed with a meningioma. A meningioma is usually benign, although in some cases can become malignant, and can usually be cured with surgery. It is a tumor originating from the meninges, or lining that covers the brain and spinal cord. 15% of all brain tumors, and 25% of all primary spinal cord tumors, are meningiomas. After some time after her initial surgery, a whisper of new growth was detected, at which time Fume chose an experimental drug, which she is still on.

While having dinner with a friend, at one point I was wiping my mouth with a napkin, and noticed that part of my upper lip had a slight numb sensation. Later, I discovered that this sensation covered a larger area, but only on half of my face and part of my head. I also noticed that when the wind was blowing, I would feel it on just half of my face.

My internist thought that it could be the result of some temporary nerve damage. I decided to watch it for a while. After some time had passed, the sensation spread rather than improve. I also started to experience periodic, momentary hearing loss from my right ear. An MRI was scheduled "just to rule things out." The tumor showed up—the size of a walnut. I was horrified. Fortunately it was benign, but it needed to be removed.

In the next week, I met with a neurosurgeon to discuss and set a date for surgery. Shortly thereafter, I caught a cold, and they could not perform surgery until I was better. During the interim, I thought I would make appointments with other doctors to get other opinions. With each appointment, I had my MRI studies under one arm and a notebook with questions in the other. I did choose a different doctor.

There were many things that needed taking care of before surgery and during the recuperation period. I planned out a detailed list, and I also made an appointment with an attorney to make out a will.

As the day of surgery drew closer, I became nervous. A friend was with me one day, and I expressed that I worried about how I would be after surgery. He said, "Maybe you'll be nicer."

Early the next morning at the hospital, I lay on the stretcher waiting my turn for surgery. I was so anxious by time they wheeled me into the operating room I was sitting straight up; however, once the anesthesiologist injected the anesthesia into the IV. The next thing I knew I was in the recovery room waking up. They immediately wheeled me into I.C.U. where I started vomiting from the anesthesia.

I also found it difficult to focus my eyes, my coordination was off, I couldn't stand without holding onto someone or something. I had significant hearing loss in my right ear, and I felt a considerable degree of numbness in the right side of my head, including the inside of my mouth. I experienced no head pain, but a muscle in my neck was very sore from the awkward position they placed my head during surgery. Every now and then I felt (and still do) a buzzing sensation on half of my tongue; and at other times, a flash of a mild pain in areas of the right gums and teeth.

After a couple of days in I.C.U., I moved to a regular unit where I remained about five days, until I transferred to another hospital for one week of rehabilitation. In total, I was off work several months mainly due to the balance problem, which improved very slowly, then eventually leveled off.

As a monitoring procedure, they scheduled me for an MRI every six months, followed by a doctor's visit. Everything remained stable until the MRI of January 1993. I received a phone call from my doctor, and he indicated that the MRI showed a whisper of new growth on the residual tumor. (The entire tumor could not be removed because of its location). He listed various options for me to think about before my appointment with him: the new gamma knife radiation, conventional radiation, or additional surgery.

During the doctor's visit and after discussing the conventional options he offered, I brought up the subject of

RU-486. I had been following this new drug because apparently some earlier studies have shown that, although it is not a cure, this drug may have an effect on the growth of some meningiomas. At this time, it is not an approved drug for use in the U.S. However, my doctor indicated that there might be a study going on and gave me a contact name and phone number.

Subsequent to several phone calls, I was finally able to start the participation process. It's a double-blind study; and yes, there are risks involved, so I had to weigh the potential side effects against the possible benefits. After starting the program, however, I may stop at any time for whatever reason. The study will last for two years, during which I will have scheduled doctor visits, MRIs, and other tests.

During the course of the study, if an MRI does show new growth, they break the code to reveal what I had been taking. If I was on the placebo, I then have the opportunity of trying the RU 486. If I had been taking the actual drug, then I will have to reconsider the original options: radiation or more surgery with radiation to follow.

On April 6, 1993, at 5 PM, I picked up the prescription. At 5:01, I took the first pill.

It's now September and I'm into the fifth month of the study. I still experience all of the symptoms I had before, but I'm hopeful that eventually RU-486 will keep the tumor at bay, and there will be no additional surgery or radiation in my future.

Patients Tell How They Cope

In the meantime, however, I try to keep informed on other possible forms of treatment, both conventional and alternative. I have also joined a support group where I have met and talked with many courageous people whose lives have been altered much more than my own. At the meetings, our $1\frac{1}{2}$ hours are oftentimes too brief as we openly share moments of joy, as well as the difficult times. For all of us, I wish continued strength as we search for a cure.

Life Is Like Climbing a Mountain:

Chris's Story

Chris was raised in Billings, Montana. She works in the garment industry as a buyer and likes running, biking, snow skiing and collecting spoons. She was diagnosed with a low-grade astrocytoma, has had two subsequent surgeries, radiation, and chemotherapy, one after the tumor recurred six years after her first surgery. She also had surgery to reduce seizures. She recently married and lives with her husband in the San Francisco Bay Area.

I was out running along the Marina Green in San Francisco on a beautiful Wednesday night in November of 1987, when I became suddenly ill. I thought my headset was shorting and I was being electrocuted. I had this buzzing, tingling feeling going through my body. I stopped, took off my headset and looked around. Nothing. I was sick to my stomach and sort of wobbly, so I sat down on the running trail. Some runners stopped to ask me if I needed help and I said yes. They flagged down some surfers who gave me a ride home—or at least that's where we were headed.

I awoke in Letterman Hospital in the Presidio after

having a grand mal seizure. My memory was blurry as to who I was, where I had been, but after some time it all came back to me. I was given seizure medications and told to see a neurologist. I did. I had an MRI and was told I had a bruise on my brain or meningitis but here's some medicine. By Christmas, I got a second opinion and was told the same thing. I had a 1% chance of having a brain tumor—if I had a brain tumor, I would be sicker!

In the first week of January 1988 I went to New York on a business trip. My second day there, I became violently ill with petit mal seizures and not knowing what was wrong with me! Fear took over. I was rushed to the hospital in New York, my films in San Francisco were flown there, and the next day I was told I had a brain tumor and needed surgery!

So in two months, I went from a 1% chance of having a brain tumor to surgery. My friend in San Francisco researched and discovered UCSF, in my back yard, was a good place to be treated for a brain tumor, so I was flown home. I had several appointments to see Doctors, but I became extremely ill with uncontrolled, non-stopping seizures that I was again rushed to the hospital. After three and a half more days of nonstop seizures, they finally subsided. I then waited in the hospital for surgery.

My surgery was successful in removing a golf ball size tumor of low grade astrocytoma. It was benign, but

I also had 6 weeks of radiation. My bald, scared head survived hair loss from radiation with scarves and a wig.

I resumed my health regimen as soon as possible, because Bay to Breakers was in May and I was going to run! Five months after my surgery I ran the world's largest fun-run and finished—I was very proud of myself because I felt I was coming back to who I was before the brain tumor. This time around, I was stronger!

My family and friends have been very supportive and understanding of my struggles and recoveries with a brain tumor. Participating in the support group is also very rewarding.

In 1993, my seizures returned, except now they were occurring sometimes every hour all day long. My physician didn't seem to think this was of concern. In my disbelief, I decided to change physicians, and find someone who would be my partner and find out what was wrong. I did find that person, and it turned out that my tumor had returned. Again I went into surgery, once for the tumor, and then again for the seizures. That was followed again by chemotherapy.

It has been one year and there is no sign of the tumor and my seizures have been reduced to a minimum. I credit this new doctor for being by my side and willing to believe me and in me.

In 1993, I also met my future husband. We recently returned from Spain where we celebrated my end of chemotherapy, and next May we will be married. You could say it has been some year!

Getting a brain tumor is frightening. Our brains are very mysterious—it's easy to accept a broken arm, but a brain tumor? I tell other patients that they've got to unload from time to time. I like being available for other patients on the telephone support network because it's nice to pick up the phone and have someone ask me, "how did you deal with this? What do you do about that?

I spoke to a woman in Iowa who hadn't been out of her bathrobe in months. She told me that her friends don't come visit her. I replied, "Well, who wants to visit a sick woman in a bathrobe? I shared with her my philosophy of recovery and told her to think of life as a mountain that you've got to climb just a little bit every day. One day she called me and said, "Guess what? My friends and I are going out! I was so happy for her I started crying.

I realize it takes a little bit of encouragement and support to climb that mountain. I feel like I got another shot at life and I want to help other people get through a tough time.

Friends Pleaded With Me to
Go to the Doctor: Julie's Story

Julie C. Arlinghaus lives in San Francisco, where she is a park ranger.
In her spare time she likes to read and is relearning calligraphy. In
June of 1992 she had surgery for a juvenile pilocytic astrocytoma.
This kind of tumor is termed a low grade glioma because it is very
slow growing and usually can be cured with surgery alone. It can be
treated with radiation or chemotherapy alone if it occurs in a part of
the brain where surgery would be impossible, such as the optic chi-
asm. It occurs most often in children and infrequently in adults, in
the area of the cerebellum. It can affect muscle coordination.

My tumor was a juvenile pilocytic astrocytoma. It was
located in my right cerebellum, and, as it grew, took away
my fine motor control, balance, and coordination. It had
grown to a diameter of six centimeters before surgery
removed it.

The tumor apparently started to grow around the time
I graduated from college, in June of 1991. I would sur-
mise that stress played no small role in its growth. After
leaving school I was no longer on the school's medical
insurance, or on my father's, and since I had very little

money I did not buy into any for a long time. Not having insurance was a major factor in my not getting medical care until very late.

In November of that year my handwriting started to become even sloppier than usual. It was difficult to control my hand: I could concentrate on its movement, but still not be able to control it. I became frightened, and retreated into myself. I did not want to run up huge medical bills I couldn't pay, and I hoped my problems would go away. Even now I know intellectually that my symptoms must have gotten worse, but I don't remember this: as my job required no writing I could ignore the deterioration and still earn a living. Being a wage-earning, productive member of society was of paramount importance to me.

I began to type my checks or even have friends write them out. I started to withdraw even more. The protective layer I built around myself in those months is still here, nearly ten months after the surgery. I am slowly tearing it down.

My friends and family pleaded with me to go to a doctor, and I kept saying that I would, but I didn't go. Besides being afraid of the bills, I think I enjoyed the attention. In January of 1992 (the Queen of England's *annus horribilis;* I knew Lizzie and I had something in common besides good looks) my boyfriend of five years moved out to San Francisco. He needed attention because this was the first time he had lived more than two hours away from home, and I was his entire support system. I was hardly the ideal support system. We broke up, got back together, and were together when I finally got insurance and went in to a doctor to see what was wrong.

I went to the public clinic at San Francisco General Hospital, and got an MRI. The neurologist I had seen there told me that it was a tumor, and that evening I was in the hospital. Five days later, on June 23, 1992, I had my surgery. I had no radiation therapy or chemotherapy, and very few physical manifestations of my tumor. I had long hair, and now it is short, but the popular styles make you look like you've had brain surgery anyway.

I had physical therapy and occupational therapy. They were not too difficult, but I was not a very dedicated student. I was not very good at being responsible for myself, I still wanted to be a child. I would not do the "homework" I was assigned, I ate junk food, I watched movies and moped.

I returned to work part-time about three weeks after the surgery, and full-time two weeks later. This was a job I loved, and love. I am a park ranger at the San Francisco Maritime National Historical Park. Ever since October of 1991 when I moved out to San Francisco I had been volunteering at the park, and when a position as a ranger opened up I applied and got it. I had been working there for two weeks when I went in for surgery, and wanting to be back was a big reason I returned to work so soon.

Patients Tell How They Cope

In September I went on training on a sailing ship for two weeks (your tax dollars are not just for bombs!). I went aloft in the middle of the night and climbed to the far end of the yard to furl sail, I went out on the bowsprit at the front of the vessel to tar the lines and to furl sail, I climbed the rigging out at sea in the dark in windy conditions. My parents nearly had a heart attack. I can't say I loved it, or that I forgot for very long about my surgery. But I did do it and I didn't fall.

The trauma of that period of my life continued after training. When I returned from sea, two things happened: my household broke up in a very nasty way, and I found out that I was pregnant. I felt like my life would never be peaceful. Two of my three housemates moved out, and now 2-$^1/_2$ wonderful people (well, two people and a cat) have far more than replaced them. Abortions are legal and accessible in San Francisco, and I took advantage of this.

November and December were actually pretty dull in comparison to the previous year, but I was feeling 1992's psychological toll. I finally went to see a psychotherapist as well as to the brain tumor support group regularly, which I probably should have been doing since June.

My tumor was far more of a psychological challenge that a physical challenge. Most of my control of my right side is back, and I'm working on my handwriting. I used to do calligraphy, and am planning on doing it again.

Navigating Through a Strange Land

My challenge was and is learning to take personal responsibility for something that I didn't ask for, but that happened anyway. It is learning the difference between "responsibility" and "fault."

"It's a Cruel, Crazy, Beautiful World:" Chris's Story

Chris deJong was diagnosed with a glioblastoma multiforme, also known as astrocytoma grade III, or high-grade glioma, the most aggressive and common form of primary brain tumor. These tumors grow rapidly, and contain cells that are very malignant. He underwent surgery and then radiation and chemotherapy. His tumor recurred six months after surgery and he has entered into another phase of surgery and gamma knife treatment, as of April, 1994. Chris was recently elected Phi Betta Kappa at the University of Oklahoma, where he is a Junior. His family lives in South Africa.

My mother was born and raised in Oklahoma. Her mother was born in "Pontotoc County, Indian Territory." My father, a South African, was recruited by the University of Oklahoma on a swimming scholarship. They met in the geology school at OU and were married in Norman. They then moved to South Africa where I was born and lived unti! 1990. I hold an American passport and dual citizenship. Like most people with experience outside the country I cherish my American passport.

Navigating Through a Strange Land

Two weeks prior to brain surgery and diagnosis with a deadly cancer I was in one hundred percent physical condition. In the middle of April, 1993, I began experiencing severe headaches. Nonprescription pain relievers were not very effective. These terrible headaches seemed to come and go but were most painful in the afternoon. I also began feeling slightly run down. Knowing that I had been exposed to mononucleosis (glandular fever) two or three weeks prior to that, I was not overly concerned about these symptoms since I thought I had contracted a case of mono.

The headaches seemed to be connected with deja vu like memories I was having. I would have a memory come into my mind which was totally unrelated to anything I had been thinking. These memories were not very powerful, just unusual. I would be suddenly reminded of an event or something specific that I had done five, six, or even ten years before. My mind would retrieve accurate memories at inappropriate times. There was nothing in my consciousness that could have reminded me of the event recalled.

Wednesday, April 28th, 1993 was the first day that anyone could possibly have known that something was wrong with me. This was the day that I actually began showing signs of altered behavior. I attended class as usual but cannot recall being there. I temporarily lost the ability to remember things, but not stored memories. Although I do not remember very much of what occurred on that day, I know I was on campus because I have an enrollment form for a summer course and notes from class dated April 28th. This later became the subject of some confusion when I tried to enroll in the class again, not remembering that I had done so already.

I was obviously in a lot of pain at this point because I went to the Health Center on campus complaining of "terrible headaches." Norgesic, a powerful headache tablet, was prescribed. I do not remember this but found the tablets in my book bag weeks later, and that visit to the health center is indicated on my charts. I saw the doctor sometime in the morning but was obviously coherent enough not to alarm anybody as to the severity of what ailed me. That morning I was tested for mono once again, thinking that the disease had finally manifested itself after a long incubation period. Of course, the test came back negative.

I took my headache tablets and apparently went about my normal campus business. I went to an appointment that I had with an OU football coach at the athletic office. I made the appointment to talk to the kicking coach about using my rugby skills in football to walk on as a kicker. I only have very brief recollections of that interview. I cannot recall talking to the kicking coach at all, but I have one clear memory of seeing Gary Gibbs, the OU head football coach, in the athletic office. Those memories are not unlike waking the day after being very drunk with only snippets of information about the previous night. Most of what happened is forgotten but some events can be recalled, usually prompted later by others who have consumed less.

From what I have been able to piece together from my friends, I must have been acting strangely, yet somehow I managed to go about regular campus business for the rest of the day. I spoke to Admiral Crow's secretary that morning. I am not sure why I went up to the Admiral's office, or if I needed to be there. From what I said and did there, Darla thought that I was "fooling around." I stayed on campus but there is no way of knowing what I did the rest of the afternoon.

What is certain is that I became incoherent and was almost incapacitated by headaches by evening. I made my way once again to the health center and was seen by a doctor at 7PM. According to the nurses, I had no idea how I had arrived there, nor could I tell them very much about myself. I had an excruciating headache and was very confused. The center staff thought that I was either critically ill or on drugs. Either way, it was determined that I needed more extensive treatment than could be provided there.

Jim, my friend, arrived to pick me up and take me to the hospital. He saw to it that I was admitted to Norman Regional Hospital. The neurologist ran a CAT scan and MRI. I was diagnosed as having a "lesion in the right temporal lobe" of my brain. Layperson's translation: I had something abnormal and unidentifiable (about the size of a lemon) in my head.

Patients Tell How They Cope

I was told that I would definitely need surgery but that the operation would have to wait until some of the swelling had gone down. The doctor said they were not sure what it was yet but that it was either a tumor or an abscess of some sort. Whatever it was, it had resulted in an enormous amount of swelling in the area that was causing my pain and confusion. I can deal with pain, but it was terribly frightening to feel my mind slipping and I could feel that. I am now convinced that 'fear of the unknown" is not only a reality but the worst of all fears.

I was given massive doses of cortical steroids in order to reduce the swelling. I became lucid and coherent, although my recollection of all of this is, of course, very hazy. My short term memory was damaged temporarily. I have never lost any stored memories, only the ability to store new ones. I was given anti-seizure medication and pain relievers, but in limited amounts because drugs might have hidden other, more serious symptoms than pain.

In the skull, swelling has nowhere to go, so it is often the build up of fluid from swelling and the resultant pressure against the various part of the brain that causes problems and/or call attention to the primary problem—called "mass effect." From my brain scans, this is evident, because even the line between the two hemispheres is bowed out to the left as a result of the edema in the temporal lobe. The doctor later said that if he had only seen the scans, and not me—drifting in and out of lucidity—

he would have assumed that I was either comatose or dead. No wonder I had headaches! I was in pain, somewhat confused, but I still managed to share jokes with my friends and family.

I have brief, fleeting recollections of events prior to, and just after the surgery, but there are some things which I do remember with amazing clarity. I remember actually fighting it, using all my inner strength against a deadly foe. I know that if I had given up that fight for a second, I would have died that night. I also remember knowing that to give up would have been much easier than to fight. I have never been afraid of death. It's just that I feel I still have a lot to accomplish and am having too much fun doing it to give up now. It is against my personal philosophy to give up anything if there is even the faintest glimmer of hope.

I have read a great deal about the mind/body connection and most contemporary literature recognizes that the psyche has enormous power over physiology. However, reading *Living Beyond Limits*, Dr. David Spiegel, has helped me to clarify where I stand in terms of the mind/body debate. Spiegel mentions the work of Dr. Bernie Siegel that suggests positive thinking and a will to live are almost as effective in battling life threatening disease as is medical science. The down side of this being, however, that it can lead patients to blame themselves for the disease and to look for ways to change their lives as sufficient therapy. And then if patients do suffer a recurrence of their disease, they will blame themselves again thinking that they must have not been concentrating hard enough or that subconsciously they want to die anyway.

Spiegel's research showed that participation in a support group can increase the survival time of patients compared to those who do not participate in a group therapy. The group therapy approach that he has been led to espouse is very similar to that described in Alcoholics Anonymous extremely successful recovery program.

I find myself drawn to both theories, but find that intellectually, for me, it makes the most sense to stick with medical science and treat the disease, not the patient. I have never denied the existence of the cancer, never tried to wish it away either. I think that I would be able to deal with it effectively again if it does recur, although I hope I never have to face the issue again, of course.

The night before the surgery was particularly bad especially since they could not administer pain killers. The nurses paged the neurologist and the brain surgeon so often that night that they considered doing an emergency surgery. Instead, some other operations were rescheduled in order to get me into surgery early on Monday morning (May 3, 1993).

Before the surgery, the neurosurgeon had warned me that I could lose some cognitive functioning as a result of such an operation, the tumor being located near areas of the brain that are responsible for memory, emotion and left motor functioning. I later joked that if I had lost all left motor functioning I would have been ALL RIGHT! When I talked to my roommate about the possibility of sustaining damage to my brain in surgery, I told him I was concerned for society if a man with my libido became a vegetable due to an operation. He agreed that a vegetable with my libido would, indeed, be a "dangerous carrot!"

Humor has sustained me throughout the ordeal, and I hope that I never lose the ability to laugh at myself and my problems. Many people were shocked by my willingness to joke about such a terrible problem, and would even scold me for being flippant or blasé. To them I would say: "This is my cancer, and I'm going to laugh about it, go get your own disease!" Naturally, I related best to the doctors and staff who felt the same way. I asked my neurosurgeon if I could save him a job by shaving my head before the surgery. His reply was that he would do it, being a "full service doctor." He is obviously a funny man, with a great attitude, he left me in stitches...!

During a five hour long craniotomy on May 3rd, the doctor removed 90-95% of the golf ball size tumor, as well as a section of the right temporal lobe from my brain. The operation was successful and my condition improved immediately. I was conscious and clear headed immediately after coming out of anesthesia. There was no long term damage, or change of any kind to my memory, emotion or motor functioning. But it did take a while for my short term memory to return to normal. I think it is 100% now, although whenever I do forget something, I am very hard on myself about it. As a result, my memory has probably improved!

The lab report indicated that the tumor was a glioblastoma multiforme, an extremely aggressive kind of malignant tumor that kills most people within six months to a year of diagnosis. Mine was the most malignant (a grade IV). I asked the doctor for a second opinion, to which he replied that I was also very ugly!

At least I knew what it was now. I was afraid while uncertainty reigned, but now I could face my fear since it was no longer an unknown 'enemy.' In many ways, knowing that I had a brain tumor was a relief. At least my confusion and pain had been physiologically, and not psychologically, caused. As for the high mortality rate associated with diagnosis of glioblastoma, I felt inclined to agree with Disreaeli: "There are three kinds of lies: lies, damned lies and statistics."

I have had alcoholism in remission for more than three years now. Successfully halting the progress of that insidious terminal disease has certainly been of assistance to me in dealing with this one. As for having not just one terminal disease but two, I have never asked: why me? I have reaped so many positive rewards from adversity, that I ask: why not me? Why not someone young and healthy like me who has a chance of fighting it.

Navigating Through a Strange Land

At the time of my hospitalization I was enrolled in a full load of classes at the University of Oklahoma. I was lucky that I got sick at the very end of the semester since all I missed was the final week of classes and exam week. Three of my professors came to visit me in the hospital. Knowing that I am a serious student, and, I suppose being reassured that I was not malingering, they each decided to excuse me from the final. So I made straight 'A's without taking any finals! Even the President of the university wrote a note to me in the hospital telling me not to worry about academic matters, and just to get well because "the University of Oklahoma wants you back in the classroom as quickly as possible!" Throughout the entire ordeal the staff and faculty at OU could not have been more accommodating. I will always be grateful for the way in which I was treated by everyone. After surgery I took the summer class that I had enrolled in before my operation.

The postoperative brain scans were inconclusive. I thought that if there was any residual tumor, it had shriveled up and died, recognizing that it had been messing with the wrong man all along. Positive thinking, a healthy attitude and humor have been implicated in cases of spontaneous remissions, or 'well behaved diseases', as doctors call it. Either way, I am determined to enjoy my life, especially if I am not destined to live out my "four score and ten" years. Why let things weigh so heavily on me? I would much rather be remembered for dealing with cancer in the way that I have chosen to than to shrivel up and die long before my heart stops beating!

All of my physicians were extremely capable and I do not think that I could have received better care anywhere in the world. However, there are some vast gaps in our scientific understanding of cancer. For example, none of the doctors could say how long the tumor had been there, where it originated and why, or what it might do next, if anything. They would frown and shake their heads and say, "it's just bad luck." Sounds like a pretty soft science to me! But medicine has made incredible advances. Everybody has an encouraging story about somebody who has beaten cancer.

Norman is just a small university town, but the local hospital has all the latest surgical equipment, and a fine department of nuclear medicine. Still, the risks involved in neurosurgery are high. One slip or miscalculation could have cost me my life, or my sight, or the use of my left arm or a change in my emotional composition or personality.

Despite the success of the surgery, some microscopic cancer cells may have been missed by the surgeon's laser scalpel or ultrasound pen. So it is standard practice to have post operative radiation and chemotherapy, especially since this kind of tumor has the ability to double its size every 10-15 days.

I was prescribed a chemotherapy called Hydroxeurea. This is not a very powerful poison but instead, is a 'radio sensitizer" which makes cancer cells more susceptible to radiation. I would take a Hydroxeurea pill 4 times a day, every other day. Chemo is a poison that attacks all fast growing cells in the body, without discrimination between cancerous and healthy cells. Cancer cells are unable to heal themselves as effectively as healthy tissue. The day in between doses would give the other healthy fast growing cells in my body (like those that line the stomach and whose loss results in nausea) time to recover. While healthy cells recover, the cancerous ones do not. So I did not suffer from any of the terrible side effects that one hears about.

Radiation was easy and painless. Radiation therapists would line me up with laser crosshairs, so that the gamma rays were beamed at exactly the right spot, in order to damage as few of the healthy brain cells as possible. I would take great pains to remind them that I could ill afford to spare any! Then they would all scamper out of the room - very encouraging! The machine would buzz for about three minutes, first on the left and then on the right side of my head. Thereafter, I would get up and walk out, totally unaffected, no pain, not even discomfort. The whole treatment lasted a mere ten to fifteen minutes, daily.

Apart from feeling a little tired, I lost hair in the areas that were irradiated. I still have two bald spots just above both ears. In order to try and impose some order on my strange hair style, I shaved the sides, and shortened the back, leaving spikes on top. This is the standard U.S. Marine Corps haircut, commonly known as a "high and tight." (Of course, I also had a huge scar on my head that looked like an enormous question mark). I was never bothered by the way I looked, though. I saw the hair loss more as an indication of the effectiveness of the radiation than as a negative side effect.

My family has been wonderful. My parents and three of my five siblings were able to be with me during the operation and afterwards as I recovered. My mother and father had planned to be in the States during the month of May, as had my eldest sister, Renee—all on business. Denise, however, left her four children with her husband, P.J., to be here with me. My brother, Mike, came down from Denver, and spent the whole night with me prior to the surgery. He was fighting it right along with me, and shared my pain. I am closer than ever to my family and friends. When I finally did fly back to South Africa in July, it was great to see Tony and Michelle, my brother and sister who were unable to come over here although it sounds like they both had to be physically restrained to prevent them from doing so.

My friends in South Africa were obviously concerned for me, knowing only that I had undergone surgery for partial removal of a cancerous brain tumor. They got together and raised enough money to fly me home! So I flew to South Africa, on July 17, for five weeks. It was, of course, wonderful to see them all, and my family, especially since most people were surprised at how well I was doing. Throughout my ordeal, I have been amazed at how lucky I am to have such wonderful, caring friends and, of course, family.

I returned to Oklahoma in August in time for the Fall semester.

I do, of course, reflect on my 'having cancer,' although not as much as I would have thought. Knowing the negative effects of being unhappy and the positive therapeutic value of a good attitude has probably made me a more positive person overall because I make a conscious effort to be happy. Like Dostoevski: "I dread only one thing, that I may not be worthy of my sufferings."

I probably get depressed about trivial things like money (or lack of it!) more often than I do about the fact that I have a cancer which, according to statistics, kills people within a year of diagnosis. I do not really mean to say that financial problems are trivial, though, since, at one point, I owed the hospital about thirty thousand dollars! While I do not include myself in this statistic, one thing I have learned from all of this is that there are no guarantees in life. In one year if I am not alive and healthy it may be because I got hit by a truck, instead of struck by this disease. I may have this disease, but as yet the disease does not have me. "Survival is the triumph of stubbornness" (Derek Walcott: *The Antilles: Fragments of Epic Memory*).

I do think that since my surgery I have become a better person; more humane, caring, kind and sensitive.

Patients Tell How They Cope

There's nothing like a brush with death to make you realize what you DO have. This is not the first time I have been struck by this though. In 1986, when I had a near fatal car accident while driving drunk at Midmar Dam, a resort near my hometown in South Africa, I fractured a vertebra in my lower back (as well as six other bones, 100 stitches, etc.). After three days in ICU I moved into an orthopedic ward. The man in the bed opposite to mine had broken the same vertebra in his back that I had, but he will never walk again. One should always take stock of what one DOES have.

I have taken to appropriating quotes from various people and media to sum up what I think about life and how I feel. After all, Winston Churchill said "It is a good thing for an uneducated man to read books of quotations." Here is one of my favorites: Johnny Clegg: "Its a cruel, crazy, beautiful world." However, the true nature of what it means to be human, it seems to me, is best described by the spirit of Ubuntu—a Xhosa proverb which goes: "Ubuntu ungamntu ngabanye abantu ." What it means is that each individual's humanity is ideally expressed through his relationship with others, and theirs in turn through a recognition of his humanity. In other words, people are people through other people. That, to me, is what life means.

I am obviously very happy that my intellectual capacities have not been affected by the surgery or radiation therapy. However, something that was very frustrating for me was that I had great trouble staying awake in the afternoons and in the evenings for several months. Sometimes I would fall asleep at my desk while I was studying. Reading on my bed was impossible. I managed to keep up academically, and all indications are that my intellectual functioning is unhindered. I love to study and enjoy my courses. The success I have enjoyed has been more a by-product of my interest than aptitude. "Success, like happiness, cannot be pursued: it must ensue and it only does so as the unintended side-effect of one's personal dedication." (Victor E. Frankl).

I dropped the dosages of the steroid and anti-seizure medication (Dilantin) which I had been on for seven months. Dilantin is a powerful drug that depresses mental activity in an attempt to prevent a seizure from occurring. Well, I have never had a seizure and so I don't think I will have one anytime soon. I can happily report that my mental activity is as good as it ever was, I think. The terrible problem I was having staying awake disappeared and I am back to normal in that regard. I am just about back to normal. However, "normal" is a relative term, and in my case, defined pretty loosely!

I will be attending the National Brain Tumor Foundation's conference for patients, families and professionals in San Francisco, in March, 1994 in order to exchange hopes and fears with fellow survivors. I feel compelled to learn as much as I can about my condition, but also to encourage others to be strong in their recovery.

Patients Tell How They Cope

I saw the conference advertised in an issue of Search, the foundation's newsletter, and applied for financial assistance from them. On the basis of my letter to them describing my situation as a university student and survivor, they funded most of my travel and accommodation. I am responsible for registration and conference fees. The clincher is that my mother and father have insisted upon paying this sum!

On February 17th I had a check up with my doctor and a brain scan. The best result I could have hoped for... it was inconclusive! MRI scans are not accurate enough to be able to say conclusively that there is no chance of the cancer recurring, and that is what my doctor told me. I picked up those films at the hospital in order to take them with me to San Francisco to the conference. At that time, I managed to buttonhole a radiologist and we sat down for a while and studied them. This meeting gave me a different perspective on the progress of the disease entirely! According to the doctor who read my films, there is "significant change with abnormal signal intensity and mass effect throughout the entire right temporal lobe and extending into the parietal lobe with marked non uniform contract enhancement highly suggestive of recurring neoplasm." Hardly the picture my neurosurgeon had painted after looking at the films and the report. I wanted to get the radiologist's report so that I could discuss my prognosis with doctors at the conference.

Navigating Through a Strange Land

I am (as you have no doubt guessed) not an active member of any Church, but I am a member of the "Episcopal Community" on the campus of the University of Oklahoma. Why? Because several years ago while working at a restaurant I waited on Friar Don, the university chaplain. We got to chatting, and since there is no Anglican Church in Norman he took me under his spiritual wing. Friar Don has been sending me the Episcopal newsletter ever since. Something that he wrote in Chaplain's Corner this month really caught my eye because of its relevance to my continuing battle with cancer.

"From the Talmud comes the saying, "Whoever saves one life, saves the world entire." The Talmud's wisdom and clear sounding of truth strikes a chord in us. It is seldom on a grand scale that we are called to live. It is a little at a time. But that little makes a great difference in the scheme of things."

What it Means To Be Human:

My Story

I was diagnosed in 1984 as having a prolactinoma; a hormone-secreting pituitary tumor. I had the transphenoidal surgery and the entire tumor was removed because it was encapsulated by calcium. I have had no recurrence of the tumor. My symptoms included ammenorria (or lack of a menstrual period) and erratic mood swings, which increasingly got worse.

In October of 1981 I set out to visit a friend in London, England. Having also obtained a six month work visa, I was prepared to stay for a least this amount of time. Before leaving a physician advised me to go on birth control pills since I was on an irregular two month cycle. I was against this, though he thought it would straighten things out. But, after taking the birth control pills, I stopped menstruating entirely. I was told by friends that it was probably just the stress of travelling and being in a new and very different environment.

By February of 1982, I had left England and was living in Spain. I still hadn't menstruated, even though it had now been six months. It was around this time that I also started noticing changes in my personality. I would burst out in anger at things that previously wouldn't have bothered me, I would weep at things only slightly sentimental or nostalgic. I felt very anxious a lot of the time, even though there was nothing to feel anxious about.

Even my thoughts seemed crowded, rushed, and unorganized. One day I remember writing over and over, "Why am I so emotional about everything?" "Why is my mind racing so much?" And, "Why do I feel anxious all the time?" This just wasn't like me. Unfortunately I lost that journal; whomever picked it up must have thought I was really cracking up. I was so disgusted at the way I felt emotionally, and having to deal with something I couldn't place or name was maddening.

But I was not willing to give up my travels, so I imagined my body as not connected to me and hoped these feelings would go away with time. I subverted the unpleasant things and focused on the good things. This was my time to live the 'bohemian life' as it were, living with several artists in a large flat spending my days drawing in the streets. I loved the richness of sights, sounds, colors and moods of the city. February always floods me with memories of blue skies, hot days, and the beautiful parks I frequented.

But by the time I had moved to San Francisco a year later, after working in Germany and San Diego, I was still having the same problems, only they were getting increasingly worse. I had many days where I could only drag myself home after work, sit in the bath, and then go to bed. I seemed to have a dull headache that never went away and my body was always tense and tight. I also felt very bloated and even a simple jog around the block would end in failure.

I alternated between feeling very ambitious and super high energy to feeling no desire to pursue anything. My body and my mind were exhausted from fighting whatever it was. Whether real or imagined I started to feel paralyzed by all the stresses and strains of living.

Looking back I realize that I simply couldn't admit to myself that something was wrong. I wanted to be a happy, successful person, like everyone else and damn it if I couldn't just live past whatever it was. I was depressed, but like an alcoholic I couldn't ask for help.

During this time period, I occasionally covered media events as a free-lance reporter. I was covering a television conference in Los Angeles, where I met a dentist who told me that I looked like I was about to crack from tension. He thought I was grinding my teeth at night and this was causing tension in my jaws and neck and spine. He said to me quite emphatically "there's something wrong with you." I remember feeling really embarrassed, thinking, "my God, do I look that bad." I realize now that I couldn't separate the me who had something wrong from the 'intellectual/spiritual/all being me. I read it like I was somehow wrong. But, I guess you could say I finally faced up to it; I couldn't very well stay in a professional environment and have people react like that to me.

I went to a gynecologist in San Diego where my parents live, and in addition to not menstruating now for two years, he detected that I was also producing milk, and that I had a high prolactin level—200 versus 5. "Ah", he sighed, "this often indicates a pituitary tumor." "I suggest when you return home you visit the hospital and have a CAT scan done." A week later I did that. After several months of odd happenings which I won't go into here, the tumor was confirmed. I looked on the scan, a little perplexed at that little pea-sized thing, and thought to myself, "You! You are what's causing me all this grief." I wanted to cry and laugh at the same time.

Somehow the tumor in my pituitary was causing my body to think it was pregnant because I was producing estrogen but not progesterone to finally shed the eggs from the body, and my breasts were full of milk. I can now also relate that it was like having premenstrual syndrome every day for two years, and this was what caused the extreme mood swings. Although at the time it felt aggressive, like a man pumped up with testosterone and steroids. The bloating was caused by water retention, and the headaches were from pressure on the optic nerves; or perhaps just my nerves altogether.

At that point I just wanted it out. All the anger and frustration I felt over the past two years seemed to gel inside of me and I was sick of the whole thing. Presented with several options, one of which was to take bromocriptine (a drug that inhibits the growth of the tumor but doesn't make it go away) for the rest of my life, I knew immediately that I would chance the surgery. I was only 25 at the time and age is always on your side in these cases.

Pituitary tumors are better news for neurosurgeons because often they can be completely cured by the initial surgery. And in my case this was true. I was in the hospital for one week, then at home for one week. After these two weeks, I returned to work. One month to the day after surgery, I menstruated for the first time in almost two years. I also remember the acute sensation of things smelling and tasting better and things just generally being clearer.

For a month or so after the surgery I remember feeling almost ecstatic with freedom. And then for some reason I crashed into a depression. I still don't know if this was a physical reaction or emotional. Probably both.

My roommate at the time took the brunt of most of this roller coaster and tried the best she could to understand; but I'm sure it was trying. I was not aware of any place to turn for help and I was mainly focused on getting back into work. I would have liked to have taken time off and really relaxed, but it wasn't possible.

Being single at the time I didn't have the luxury of someone to lean on. I've always believed that it is easier for a married person in these circumstances because there is a second paycheck and someone to make you feel better. When you are alone, the entire burden is on you, and it's frightening and stressful. But you don't have time to dwell on the fears. I was not insured at the time and I was fortunate that my physician made it possible for me to be treated for a nominal fee. But also my pride prevented me from asking for help from my parents and my friends, and that was a mistake. One friend was so angry and hurt that I didn't tell her, and let her help me. She said, "that's what friends are for." I thought about that for a long time.

It has been ten years and there has been no recurrence of the tumor, which is typical if the entire tumor is removed (at least to their knowledge). This is not always the case, however, and for some pituitary patients, radiation is also required because some tumor is remaining. If the entire or partial pituitary is removed, then medication is necessary to reproduce the hormones which are produced by the pituitary gland, which regulates the reproductive system in women and other major functions in all people, including metabolism. The pituitary gland is called the master gland because it issues many of the hormones within the body. A tumor of the pituitary presents the most problems for children because they are still growing and it can inhibit natural growth patterns.

Of all the things I tried to do to feel normal again after dealing with hospitals and bureaucracies and the city, a move back to my home town was the thing that worked the best. When the plane started to descend over the lakes and farmland of Minnesota that I had missed so much over the years, tears welled in my eyes. "I'm home," I remember thinking, as the tears streamed down my face. "It's really over with." It was such a relief to be in a familiar and safe place.

I lived with my girlfriend in the country and worked downtown with a wonderful group of people. Every day I rode an old rickety bus for an hour-long long trip through small towns along the lake and then through the woods, which changed through the seasons from green to a kaleidoscope of color to the white of snow, and then arrived smack into downtown almost with surprise. Sometimes old friends would happen onto the bus and we'd talk all the way to work together. I was in heaven.

My friend's mother, however, was appalled at how thin I was and told her I better get fed right. Ironically, one year after I returned to San Francisco to work with the National Brain Tumor Foundation, and fatter I might add, her brother-in-law was diagnosed with a brain tumor.

One of the problems with illnesses and recovery is that it is hard to locate the source for some of our emotions and actions. Nothing happens in a vacuum. Our lives are still going on in other areas, and while we are struggling with one problem, other equally disturbing things may be going on at the same time. And this was certainly true in my case. However, I also did not grieve these other serious events until years later. If anything, I tend to minimizes things; make them seem less important. But now I know that in fact we do 'store things' in our bodies and eventually it comes out in great heaves and cries. When too many things are happening at the same time you just shut down and go on autopilot.

Many people will say, directly or indirectly, "Oh snap out of it, get back to your old self." But that's unrealistic, almost stupid and silly if you think about. That's right, I'll just go back to being..., what? Innocent? Unaffected? We don't go back to the way we were. These things change us. It's called growth, for better or for worse. Some of this is voluntary, some of it is subconsciously driven.

On the one hand, I am a much more emotional person than I used to be and I think that is probably good, but I am also much more protective of myself. I am more cautious about events that produce too much anxiety, because in that state I am reminded of how I felt all those years.

I still occasionally feel sad for that time in my life, if something reminds me of it. Doing this book caused me great inner turmoil at times. Every time I started to write my own account I'd get really depressed, although I wasn't quite sure why. At one point I quit the entire project even though it was almost done.

I cried to my friend that thinking about it made me relive how frightened I was during that time in my life; something I never let myself feel at the time. Writing is hard that way; it definitely brings things to the fore.

When I go through phases like this, feeling confused and frustrated, I find praying comforts me more than anything else. I am not a religious person in the traditional sense, I don't go to church, although I do believe in the concept of fellowship at a church. However, I have always felt a connection to a God, and believe that this faith has helped me through many things.

Later during that week I sat down in my room and out of a need to do something creative I started to draw. What came out was the basic design of the book and some other work. I was uplifted by this and after some conversations with friends I decided to finish the project. I have to tell you though writing these personal things with the thought that the public is going to read it is not easy.

When I hear the word recover, it seems that people mean they want to recoup their loss, or themselves. But to me it means to integrate and evolve, to redefine or recover what was with something new. Life is not so much linear, but a topographical map where we can overlay past terrain with new ideas and perspectives. I love traveling for this reason; it's so refreshing. So is making a new friend. We get a new start.

It's absolutely true that there is always hope for a good outcome. I am an example of that. But I also know many people who have problems for many years after their treatment. And there are attendant feelings of anger, frustration and fear for a variety of legitimate reasons. Unfortunately, many books aimed at cancer patients in the popular press only focus on the good results and gloss over a vast population who have to deal with ongoing day to day problems. And thus people who don't get better think there's something wrong with them.

Books like this perpetuate a kind of thinking in society that only the happy and healthy, the fighters and the winners are to be applauded, while pain and suffering are ugly and to be avoided at all costs. It puts shame upon people for a natural response to a bad life event. How dare they, I find myself muttering as I walk down the street.

Grief and suffering are a natural by-product of something that has gone wrong, as are feelings of exhilaration when things go right. Never be ashamed of the fact that you have a whole range of emotions. That's what it means to be human. We are not robots, after all. It's important to directly address problems and feelings that come up. Don't ignore them, rather give them full vent. Let them run their course.

However it's important to remember that there's still the essence of you inside. A creative person who wants to do the activities they have always loved. Despite what's happening it helps to continue to do those things. It provides an anchor of your old self when you feel so many new things happening. Keep doing the things you love and find some new inspiring things to try.

As an end to my story, I'd like to share two drawings

I did that express how I felt. Like many people I think of
the pursuit of art as completing something beautiful (even
though I was an art major and should know better). However, art was a perfect medium for this. The first depicts
how I felt before diagnosis, and the second is years later.

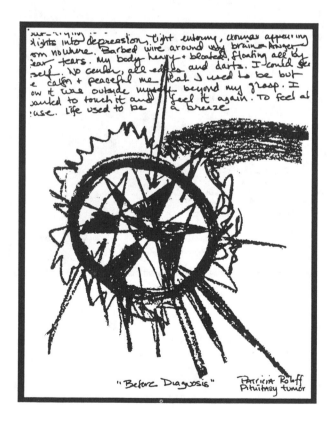

"Before Diagnosis"

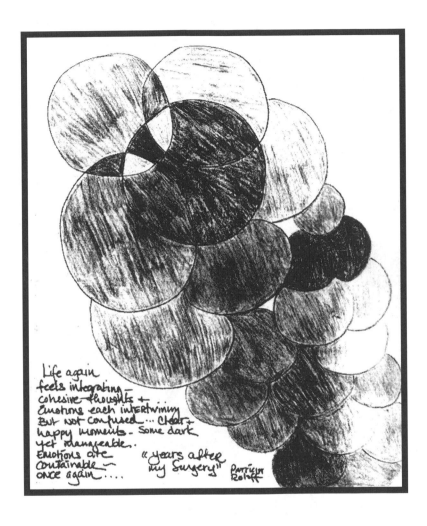

Life again
feels integrating—
cohesive thoughts +
emotions each intertwining
But not confused ... clear—
happy moments - some dark
yet manageable.
Emotions are
containable—
once again .....

"years after
my surgery"   Patricia
Roth

Creativity is a source, not an answer. It is a reflection of your inner self, not a directive from the outer world. It gives voice to the unspoken and form to the abstract. It is accessible and tangible. It heals and is the healer. It is spiritual and it is concrete. It is courage and strength, both particular and yet universal. It brings light to the darkness. It brings peace and wholeness. It reconnects what is unplugged. It is narrative medicine.

Chapter Three

Family Members Tell Their Stories

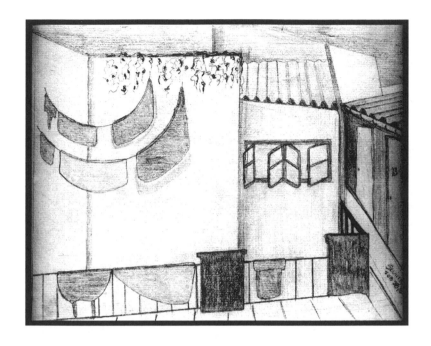

I No Longer Fear Death:

Linda's Story

This letter was written after the death of her daughter, Jamie. The entire story of Jamie, including this letter, is published in the book, To Live Until We Say Good-bye, by Dr. Elizabeth Kubler Ross and Mal Warshaw (referenced in the reading section).

In many ways, my life really began just before I learned that my daughter had a brain tumor. Most of my life before that followed a typical pattern. I went to college, taught for five years, married, became the mother of two children, and acquired a house in the suburbs. About a year before Jamie's tumor was diagnosed, I began to feel that I needed something more, something for myself. I became more involved in the parent-participating cooperative nursery school my son attended, joined a women's consciousness-raising group, and went into therapy. The growth and changes that came from these experiences may have helped to prepare me for the time ahead with Jamie but they also contributed to the end of my marriage. I was in the middle of divorce proceedings when I learned about Jamie's tumor. All of my excitement and plans for the future vanished at that moment. I knew that my own life would have to wait.

From the moment of her birth, for some reason Jamie and I shared a very special love. I knew that she would need me even more now, and I needed to be with her too. Learning about her illness began the most profound and emotionally intense time of my life. Everything that ever happened to me before belonged to another lifetime. All my energy was now centered on the fight for Jamie's life. There were moments when I resented the limitations Jamie's illness put on me, but if she was to die, I had to know I had done everything within my power for her.

I was told how serious Jamie's illness was from the beginning, for I insisted on knowing the truth. Although chances were slim that she would survive, there was room for a little hope. However, at the beginning, I found it hard to hold onto that hope. We suddenly entered an unknown yet terrifying world. The staff at Babies' Hospital helped ease the transition somewhat, but it was difficult to watch Jamie go through the brain scans and the radiation treatments. Yet she accepted it all and gave me the strength I needed. I knew that, despite my despair, I had to make every moment precious for her.

Although I was no longer married, I was not entirely alone. Throughout Jamie's illness, I had the constant love and help of my parents and friends. Although they could not completely know the depth and complexity of my feelings, they were with me, for they too needed to do whatever they could to help Jamie, my son Rusty, and myself. At times I found it difficult to relate to these people, as dear and wonderful as they were to me, precisely because this was happening to me, not to them. They could leave me and return to their more 'normal' lives while my world was shattered. Yet I know I could never have made it through Jamie's illness without them.

I experienced many moments of intense anger and bitterness. Despite the depth of my love for Jamie, there were times when I was so angry at her for putting me through this, for making me face the possibility of losing someone so precious to me, for depriving me of the chance to continue to love her and guide her and share in her growing up loved and loving. At the same time, I was aware of all she had given me in so short a time.

One of the things that made it so hard for me to face my life without Jamie was that I did not believe in any kind of life after death. I had always been terrified at the thought of my own death, believing it would mean the end of all consciousness, although I tried not to think about it and certainly never talked about it. Many of my friends do believe that there is life after death, but I rejected their attempts to talk to me about this. I did not think it would be at all comforting to me if I believed that a part of Jamie would survive death. I was more concerned with the tremendous loss I would have to cope with if she died.

Navigating Through a Strange Land

Although part of me used a great deal of denial all through Jamie's illness, I also felt a need to try to prepare myself for her death. I began to read, beginning with Dr. Kubler-Ross's *On Death and Dying*. Perhaps my experience in a consciousness-raising group led to my desire to talk to other people who were going through a similar experience. Through Hospice of Rockland, I became part of a group of relatives of cancer patients. It was with these people that I could deal with the feelings and fears that I often pushed away.

It's also through a member of this group that I met Mal Warshaw and became part of this book. I had been helped by so many people and I hoped that by sharing my experience, others would learn that they did not have to face alone the loss of their child.

I met Dr. Kubler-Ross just after I learned that Jamie's tumor was growing again and there was little that could be done for her. I was in the middle of my own investigation of possible future treatments. I could not give up, even though intellectually I knew Jamie was dying. Within a few minutes, Dr. Kubler-Ross knew exactly what I needed and, with Jamie's help, she gave it to me. She asked Jamie to draw a picture. It was Dr. Kubler-Ross's interpretation of this picture that was the first step for me in coming to acceptance of the inevitability of Jamie's death and a change in my thinking about death itself. Among the many shapes on Jamie's pictures was a free-floating purple balloon. Dr. Kubler-Ross pointed out to me that this balloon's color, position on the page, and its lack of connection to any other shape indicated that Jamie knew what was happening to her and accepted without fear the transition she was about to make. I needed to know that the future would not be difficult for her.

Dr. Kubler-Ross also knew that I was not allowing my feelings of anger and despair to surface as much as they should. A few days after her visit, she sent me a piece of rubber hose to beat against some sturdy object when I needed to get those feelings out. I have used it and it works.

We talked about a possible way of setting up my house if Jamie were ever bedridden. That time did come. I had taken Jamie to the hospital for one last treatment. It did not help and her condition steadily worsened. She needed constant and complete care but she wanted to go home. Although I was very frightened, I decided to go along with Jamie's expressed desire. Dr. Kubler-Ross visited us again during Jamie's last three weeks at home and was so supportive of what I was doing. I came to realize how much I needed that time at home with Jamie. It made it possible for me to fully accept the fact that Jamie had to die. It also gave me a chance to do all that was left to be done for her—to make her comfortable, to provide her with familiar things, and most important, to surround her with the love of her family and friends. I too was surrounded, I could never have brought Jamie home without the love and help of so many people, my parents, my friends, especially Liz, Joan, Carol, Lois, and Lee as well as many others at Babies' Hospital. All of us, including my son, shared in caring for Jamie. It was especially important for Rusty to be part of this time. He had been shut out often when I was in the hospital with Jamie or taking her there for treatments. He has some beautiful memories from those last three weeks—reading to Jamie, polishing her nails, or just sitting with her on her bed and holding her hand.

I knew I had done the right thing in bringing Jamie home, but a few days before she died, I wavered briefly in my determination to keep her at home until the end. There were medical complication I was not sure I could handle. I called Dr. Kubler-Ross, and with only a few words she gave me the reassurance I needed. At that point, Jamie was in no pain and rarely awake. Dr. Kubler-Ross strengthened my newly forming belief that Jamie's consciousness was focused elsewhere but she was still surrounded by love. I knew then that I would not take her back to the hospital. It helped me so much to know that I could turn to Dr. Kubler-Ross at any time with any problem and she would be there.

As Jamie's condition worsened, I tried to concentrate on the purple balloon and all it represented. I found myself wanting and needing to believe that part of Jamie would still exist somewhere, somehow, after her body died. During the week, despite episodes of respiratory distress, Jamie became very peaceful, and I no longer feared what was happening. I could almost see the purple balloon gently pulling on its string until at last it separated and floated away. I miss Jamie so much, but out of the pain has come much growth and learning. I no longer fear death, for as I held Jamie in my arms as she died, I saw nothing to fear. I no longer believe that death is an end. Even as I drove off from the cemetery, I had no feeling of having left my child there. She was with me as she has been many times since her death. In the midst of all the anguish are so many beautiful memories. Jamie's courage, her joy, her love will always be with me. She was truly a very precious gift."

Navigating Through a Strange Land

May My Son's Dream Come True: Bonnie's Story

Bonnie Feldman founded The Brain Tumor Society, a nonprofit foundation in Boston, Massachusetts, during the illness of her son, Seth. Seth was diagnosed with a glioblastoma multiforme at aged 14, and lived until his 18th birthday. She and her husband live outside of the Boston area. She is also former chairman of the North American Brain Tumor Coalition.

In August of 1985, my son Seth, aged 14, was diagnosed with a glioblastoma multiforme. Seth was an honor student, an avid skier, and a great fan of the British rock group, The Who. Seth played varsity tennis and freshman football at his high school, and was away at football camp when he became ill.

Given only eight months to live, Seth grappled with life and death issues while bemoaning the fact that he had planned to take a new language in school—German, and how tough it would be to catch up.

Following his initial surgery, Seth embarked on a six-week course of intensive chemotherapy requiring three hospitalizations, and five weeks of twice daily radiation treatments. As soon as he felt bored, and ready for a new challenge, we arranged for his German teacher to come to our home to tutor him. She was terrific! Following his surgery, Seth had become photophobic, and could not manage any visual concentration without a great deal of discomfort. He could not read or watch television. His memory, however, was not impaired. To help Seth learn new sounds and a new German vocabulary, his teacher made giant flash cards, which she literally flashed at him for the very briefest of moments, to enable him to visualize this new language.

Before long, we began reading Seth the books from his honors English class, secured a tape recorder for the visually handicapped, and eventually obtained a number of the assigned books on tape. By December, he was able to attend school for one period a day. When his energy increased, he went for two classes—German and English. He was very fortunate in that these two classes had been scheduled back-to-back. Seth was determined to begin his honors Chemistry program after Christmas vacation. We arranged for him to lie down in the nurses office everyday between his English and Chemistry classes.

Instead, Seth wound up back in the hospital for four weeks, suffering from massive edema as a result of the radiation treatments he had received. He had tremendous muscle wasting as a result of what his physician called "industrial doses" of Decadron (a drug used to reduce swelling in the brain), which set him back for the next few months.

I could go on and on about Seth's subsequent medical problems—his seizure disorder and the difficulty we had regulating his chemical meningitis, and a twisted neck which required traction. He lost over twenty pounds in two weeks and came home from the hospital unable to walk or care for himself in any way.

With great will and determination and rehabilitation, Seth attended his junior prom just five weeks later, and loved every minute of it. Unfortunately, he was once again experiencing new tumor growth which was affecting the strength on one side of his body. Shortly after school ended, he began a new course of chemotherapy, M.O.P.P., a protocol which had been used for years in the treatment of Hodgkin's Disease, which was then being tried, with some degree of success, for glioblastoma.

Every time Seth was cut down, he would engage, as soon as possible, in the challenge of recovery. When, because of weakness, he could do no more than lie on the couch all day, he would push himself to take a 1/2 block walk. As his energy increased, he'd plan a half-day outing. Then he'd start lifting weights or go to rehab. When he could not play football, he taught himself to be a kicker. Before long, he was back on the slopes. Even if we had to drive him to the ski lift and carry his skis for him, he would take some runs.

Family Members Tell Their Stories

Seth used what extra energy he had to speak on behalf of the institute at which he had been treated. He spoke on radiothons, at golf tournaments, and to groups of volunteers. He wanted to raise money for brain tumor research so that someday others would not have to go through what he had gone through. One day, during treatment, Seth asked me what was the worst treatment for a brain tumor. I took my best guess. His answer: "No treatment at all."

Seth viewed his illness as a hurdle to get over. He wanted only to be a normal teenager. It had been his life-long dream to attend Dartmouth College. Despite the fact that he had no energy to take the campus tours, we visited five colleges the summer before his senior year. He decided to apply to Dartmouth early decision. As a senior, he had not yet taken his College Board Exams. But that didn't stop him. He was on two successive Saturdays, resting periodically in the nurses office. He passed with flying colors and got his early admission to Dartmouth!

Seth graduated with the other members of his senior class to a standing ovation, attended his senior prom, and most amazingly, set off for college. The summer following graduation, he retrained himself to read so that he would not need a reader or a special tape recorder at school. He plowed through nine novels, the first books he had read in three years. He felt the best he had felt in three years. His doctors wanted him to go back on chemotherapy, but he refused.

Navigating Through a Strange Land

Once again, special arrangements were made at school. Seth would take two of the required three courses, live in a single room on a freshman floor, so that he could have the socialization while being able to get his much needed rest. His dormitory was located close to the library and cafeteria and the campus police could drive him to any distant classes or activities. While he was exempt from any physical education requirement, always looking for a challenge, Seth took up racquetball.

On Halloween of 1988, Seth's tumor recurred for the last time. He found himself a reader and managed, as best he could, to stay at school until final exams. In his mind, he had completed his first term. He regretted not having been able to spend more time at Dartmouth, where he had spent the happiest days of his life.

Seth passed away two weeks after he returned home, just days before his eighteenth birthday. He never lost his sense of humor or his indomitable spirit. His strength, his courage, and an abounding love of life were his legacies. Seth taught me that just about anything is possible when you set your mind to something.

While each story is unique, it seems that every parent with whom I have spoken, who has or has had a child with a brain tumor, has drawn their strength from that child. After all, as a parent, what could be worse than having your child diagnosed with a life threatening problem, and watching that child undergo treatment? Aren't we, as parents, supposed to be able to make it all better?

Instead we become our child's advocate and facilitator. It certainly helps us, when we feel we can help them. Teenagers present an unusual challenge. While their friends are gaining more and more independence, they must rely, more than ever, on their parents. That is why it is important to include them in decision making processes, whenever possible.

When Seth set off for college, I knew I would have new found time on my hands. As pointed out to me by the Directors of Development and Pediatric Oncology at the institute at which my son had been treated, there was a tremendous need for a grassroots organization to raise public awareness of the brain tumor problem and to raise critically needed funds for research.

Drawing my inspiration from Seth, I researched what other brain tumor organizations were out there, contacted the leaders of these groups, learned about the objectives of each group and how they were organized, and promised myself to someday get the leaders of these groups together to share information and to take on initiatives that no one group could accomplish individually. As there was no brain tumor organization east of Chicago or north of Atlanta, and the group in Atlanta was a locally focused pediatric group, I set out to establish The Brain Tumor Society, which would be a national organization, based in Boston. I put together a Board of Directors with expertise in a number of different areas and a deep commitment to the cause, and I recruited a group of nationally recognized physicians, highly respected for their work in this area, to participate as our Medical Advisory Board. Our mission was clear—our focus would be on fund-raising for research, education and support to patients and families.

The Society has accomplished a great deal in the past four short years. We have assisted hundreds of patients and families throughout this country and beyond. We disseminate educational information, encourage the formation of brain tumor support groups and provide those in need access to such groups. For those who cannot attend support group meetings, we have instituted a patient/family telephone network.

With the belief that education must occur on many levels, the Society not only provides patients and their loved ones with up-to-date information concerning their specific tumor types and treatment options, the Society contributes to continuing education for doctors and nurses, as well. In April of 1993, the Society cosponsored an international workshop to bring together researchers and clinicians to discuss the critical problem of Growth Control in Central Nervous System Tumors. The workshop was a resounding success, and a similar workshop will be held this spring.

Each year, the Brain Tumor Society hosts an annual meeting that is open to the public and attended by several hundred patients, family members, friends, and health professionals from six or seven different states. The theme of the evening is invariably a hopeful and inspiring one, and on this occasion we award The Brain Tumor Society Research Grants. The Society has declared as a top priority the support of innovative basic scientific research projects directed at finding the causes and cures of brain tumors.

Through the Society's Campuses Against Cancer program, college students throughout the country are raising both awareness and funds to fight brain tumors, a problem that all too frequently affects their age group. The Society uses every opportunity to generate publicity about the issue in order to bring greater public awareness to bear in this battle.

As I had promised myself early on, in February, 1990, just months after the founding of The Brain Tumor Society, the leaders of six independent brain tumor organization held their first meeting. The lines of communication were opened. In April of 1991, eight such groups located throughout the United States and Canada formed the North American Brain Tumor Coalition. I was given the honor and entrusted with the responsibility of becoming the Coalition's first Chairman.

In May of 1992, as Chairman of the North American Brain Tumor Coalition, President of The Brain Tumor Society, and a mother who had lost her son to a brain tumor, I testified before the United States House of Representatives Committee on Appropriations, Subcommittee on Labor, Health and Human Services, Education and Related Agencies as to the critical need for the establishment of brain tumor research centers. It was rumored that the funding of four centers was being taken under consideration, but that the final decision regarding numbers and figures had yet to be determined. In the fall of 1992, I received word that eight brain tumor research centers would be established at a cost of $9.18 million.

In the spring of 1993, a symposium was held in Washington, D.C. to educate the Coalition membership as to ways in which the Coalition could most effectively educate Congress and the National Institutes of Health on the importance of brain tumor research, and the critical need for increased funding to be allocated for that purpose. The Coalition plans to focus many of its efforts in this direction.

To enhance our credibility and fortify our case, the Coalition will, for the first time, be able to paint a more accurate statistical picture, drawing on information provided by the Central Brain Tumor Registry of the United States. As a member of the Board of Directors of this newly formed registry, I am greatly encouraged by our progress in this much needed area.

When Seth first left for college and I decided to volunteer my time and direct my energies to the brain tumor cause, I felt I was continuing Seth's work. When he died, I felt an overwhelming need to make something positive come from this truly devastating experience.

After all, no parent expects to bury a child. The loss of a child defies, in my mind, the natural order of life.

Today, through my work at The Brain Tumor Society, I speak to many patients and concerned family members and friends. It makes me feel a little better if I can help someone else. I am kept focused and profoundly motivated by those who are still in need. Whenever I doubt my ability to face a particular circumstance, be it a medical problem, an important meeting or a large audience, I think of Seth and his bravery and his courage, and I think, I can do that. And I do it.

It was Seth's dream that someday others would not have to go through what he had gone through. With the help of my loving and supportive husband, Sid, the blessing of our delightful daughter, Jill, and the commitment and dedication of the wonderful volunteers and professionals with whom we work, someday Seth's dream will come true.

"We Realized a Lot of Things Too Late:" Darryl's Story

Darryl's father was diagnosed with a glioblastoma and died four months later. He and his wife and children live in Kansas, where he is a physician in private practice.

My dad recently died four months after he was diagnosed with a glioblastoma multiforme. I happen to be a doctor, which has some relevance, as you'll see later, and this story is less about my dad than about his family and his care. In retrospect, we realized a lot of things too late, and they might have made our lives, and the time that he had left, better.

My dad was admitted to a University Hospital for a fever and confusion. He had a CT scan and an MRI. Our neurologist told us right up to the morning of the surgery that while this could be cancer, that he still hoped that it might be a brain abscess. I later learned that the MRI had the classic appearance of a glioblastoma, and still cannot understand why a physician could not tell another physician what was really going on. I had approached this problem as I often do, objectively, and not very emotionally. My dad's neurosurgeon described my parents as philosophical. We were hardly in danger of falling apart.

The surgery was uneventful, and the surgeon told us that the tumor was relatively small, in an accessible location, and that he got a lot of it out. Again we were quite hopeful that my dad would be with us for "some" time.

My mom, brother and I began to talk to my dad about closing his legal practice. He had worked long enough, and we all thought that he and my mom would be well off financially if he stopped working now. He had always insisted that he could not stop working because he needed more money to retire on, perhaps a result of having grown up poor during the Depression. But since no one knew how much time he would have left, we felt strongly that he should not spend it on work. He refused to consider closing his practice. His internist talked with him, but again he put this off until he had the final diagnosis.

At the time it seemed that his stubbornness was due to the denial one would expect with his diagnosis, but looking back on it, we can see that his ability to reason had already been greatly affected by the tumor. We argued about this several times, and I finally left the hospital in disgust, flying home a day earlier than I had planned, as obviously I was going to be of little use, and the pathology report on the tumor might not be back for days.

As it turned out, the neurosurgeon came to the room while I was in the cab to the airport, and gave my folks the worst news, that the tumor was of the most aggressive sort, a glioblastoma. He told my mom, but not my dad, that the average survival was 12 months. My dad knew that the news was bad, but my mom didn't feel comfortable with giving him the numbers. However, when I spoke with the neurosurgeon from the airport he clearly painted a rosy picture, saying that my father fell into a good prognostic group and would "be a good companion to my mom for perhaps three years."

Now I don't expect docs to tell the future, nor do I hold them to the length of time they give patients to live. There are all too many stories where patients outlive their doc's prediction. And one always fears shortening a patient's survival with too gloomy an outlook. However, looking on the brightest side can really have its drawbacks.

We were told that he should have conventional radiation and chemotherapy, and that no experimental protocols could be considered without having failed these. In retrospect, I would have asked for all the different protocols that were being tried in the country—by the time patients are really sick they can't be flown to distant cities, or housed in motels, or cared for by their spouses unassisted. By the time someone fails the conventional therapy, as my dad did, it may be too late to consider other options.

We pursued the traditional therapy, hopeful that he would have some response, and perhaps a few months of decent life before he relapsed. I planned to take the family on vacation in October, after he completed the radiation and recovered from its effects. He did well for six weeks but nose-dived with two weeks to go.

Every day after this proved to be an ever increasing ordeal for my mother. At first we ascribed his fatigue to the radiation therapy. But it was much more profound than this. He'd sleep for 20 hours a day, and it would take my mother hours of screaming and coaxing to get him ready for their daily trip for radiation therapy. He'd scream if you touched him, and it was impossible to do much without his cooperation, which was nonexistent. He was incontinent. He'd stay for hours in the bathroom, unable to get off the toilet, and unwilling to accept help. It would take a monumental effort to get him to eat or to take his medication. Still his behavior was assumed to be a result of the radiation treatment.

Finally the treatment was over and my family flew to spend time with my parents and my brother and my sister's family. It took us three hours to get him out of a chair in the den the first night we arrived, and the next day it took us three hours to get him into the car for the trip to my brother. We arrived in the early afternoon, but we could not get him out of the car for five hours. We alternated coaxing, talking, then screaming and cursing at him, one person relieving the other when we got out of hand, thinking that it was a matter of stubbornness, because he refused all help. Really, it was the tumor talking, because he just could not put together the many movements and decisions needed to get himself out of a car. He would start to move then lose track of what he was doing, again and again.

We realized on some level that he had changed neurologically, but didn't want to believe this was so. We still clung to the idea that it was the fatigue from the radiation. My wife finally led him into the house at nightfall, knowing that this was really the end. Unfortunately, the physicians were of no help in giving us an explanation of why this was happening. When I stressed to them how difficult it was getting to care for him, we increased his medication to decrease intracranial pressure. This seemed to help a little.

Now in all fairness, the doctors never really saw how bad he was, because once my mother finally got him up and moving, often after many hours of struggling, he was always awake and a pretty good actor for his radiation treatments and other visits. But my mom had been describing his worsening symptoms to them, and when he was scheduled for a repeat MRI and to see his neurologist again, my mom was prepared to not accept the usual pronouncement that he was doing fine and was to be seen again in two weeks.

When the neurologist said exactly that, my mom prepared for this, took his arm physically and said "doctor he is not all right. Look at him, he's much worse." He took her into the next room and told her that things were very bad, that the tumor was much larger on MRI and had not responded to radiation and chemo and that he would die soon, and that we should get a doctor near us to take care of this stage of his illness. I heard this a few hours later.

My dad had five physicians; an internist, a neurologist, a neurosurgeon, a radiation oncologist and a chemotherapy oncologist. What he needed was a doctor; someone who would contact the radiologist who read the MRI, and then determine my dad's options from the neurosurgeon, neurologist and chemotherapist. For example, was it worth the struggle to continue coming to the hospital for chemotherapy and the blood tests needed. I remarked to my wife about the trouble I was having coordinating my dad's care, in spite of the fact that I was a doc and actually knew the system. I called and asked the radiation oncologist, who was a very open and honest man, if he would be "the doctor," and he said he'd be glad to fulfill that role. After he made his calls, we decided to stop all treatment. By this time my dad could not communicate by phone, and slept most of the time.

The illness and its treatment was difficult enough for my mom, as she was sole caregiver and transporter, and because we had no idea of what was going on eight weeks after the initial surgery. But because we never had someone really tell my dad his prognosis and we hoped that he would recover for a time, he never came to grips with his business. His partners called every day for him and he'd never take the calls. He wouldn't allow us to reveal his illness, and accused us of disloyalty if we did. He told me after his radiation that he actually planned to go back to work. He was a very independent and stubborn person to the end.

My mom had to take care of him and deal with partners who screamed at her almost daily. She was terrified of answering the phone in her own house. And my phone conversations while my dad could still talk on the phone invariably ended with my arguing with him over his treatment of my mom when she'd try to discuss his practice and his need to recognize what she was going through, and that he needed to retire. My mother did not feel that she could do this without his permission.

The result of this was that all of our interactions with my dad during the middle part of his illness were negative; fighting over his getting ready for the daily treatments, over getting up to eat, over getting out of the bathroom, or physically caring for him, or about his practice and the calls he was receiving. So we never got a chance to deal positively with his illness, and certainly never got a chance to do this with him, or really say good-bye. By the time that we realized that he'd have no good time, he was too far gone to communicate with us.

To add to this, my mom had to deal with all the details of his practice after my dad died. She got a little help from her son-in-law, and she and I talked every night, but the major burden was clearly on her. This required an amount of strength and energy that my mom fortunately possessed.

This condenses and in a way trivializes the emotional trials that we experienced. My dad maintained his defenses and a considerable amount of denial, until he probably became so disoriented that his illness was not much of an issue to him. But we had real problems as a result of not really knowing at each step why he acted as he did, how his tumor was progressing, and when to step in and really deal with his affairs. My mom feels tremendous guilt now about having put him through the ordeal of treatment when it obviously did no good.

In retrospect, we should have known that his problems were largely due to his tumor, and that he was using his considerable remaining resources to cover and maintain a semblance of normality. Instead of dealing with the conflict over the issues that I mentioned, we would have liked to have spent the remaining time he had in a more positive way.

Note: Darryl is a fictional name for this author who wishes to remain anonymous.

Navigating Through a Strange Land

I Could Hardly Say the Words: My Daughter Has Cancer: Richard's Story

Richard's daughter was diagnosed with a Ganglioneuroma. She had surgery, radiation and chemotherapy, and is doing well. He wrote this story for Search when I was editor. He and his family live in the valley, east of San Francisco.

I suppose that the most important part of solving any problem is to identify it, label it, and then outline a course of action. I remember in November of 1984, the neurologist telling us, "your daughter has a deposit in the spinal ganglia of her brain. It could be a calcium deposit or maybe a cyst." He went all around the word "tumor" as if we couldn't handle it. He was almost right. It was darned hard to handle.

I came home, back to my radiator and muffler shop, and called my banker. With tears in my eyes and a shaking voice, I asked him for enough money to run the business for six months, because I knew that one of my little girls was going to need all of us by her side. God bless my banker and our small town for the support which we got.

It wasn't until early in 1985 that I finally realized the

problem and was able to say it, "My daughter has cancer." I think that I did everything I could in the first two months to avoid saying that. I kept my mind occupied with the problems, the many trips to San Francisco, the arrangements that had to be made, our younger daughter Stephanie; almost anything to keep from saying "Leslie has a brain tumor."

I'm pretty good at fixing things. It took me a long time to realize that they couldn't just cut this thing out. They couldn't just fix it.

One starts to ask the same questions that every parent asks. Why my kid? Why us? Cancer in kids is something that happens in big cities, not small town folks like us. We eat simple, eat fresh food and live healthy lives. Heck, Leslie is a class one athlete. She races an 80KX Kawasaki. She's no wimp! But you know what, cancer just doesn't care about that.

So, at this point, your family really becomes one. You tell your friends, your family, your church that you need their thoughts and prayers. You become as tough as your kid and say - and most important know - that your "pride and joy" is going to beat this problem. You learn about radiation and chemotherapy. Your dinner conversations include words and terms that you never knew existed.

You meet other people from different parts of the state, nation and world with problems that make yours look small in comparison. Then you say, "thank you Lord, for letting us handle this and steering us in the right direction." You learn to accept that some of the kids you've met might not make it. But not your kid, because you know she will. The word is attitude. You must be positive.

Well, Leslie has made it, and made it well. She was on the honor roll her entire sophomore year and also on the high school track team. Her special event is the low hurdles. She had a bad fall at the first of the season but came bouncing back at the end. She is currently Cotton Queen in Corcoran, our town. She is past Honored Queen of Job's Daughters and does an excellent job in her memory work. She conducts a meeting well and has spoken before such groups as the Chamber of Commerce of Corcoran and has received a standing ovation. When she graduated from eighth grade, she received the American Legion Award. She accepted it in a beautiful dress and almost no hair, but I don't think that anybody noticed the lack of hair.

Yes, we're proud of both our daughters. We are thankful for the strong attitudes and an amazing will to live. Leslie has a tremor remaining on her right side, not bad, but it makes for a good laugh to watch her carry drinks in her right hand. She has gone from right-handed to left, and her memory is not as great as it once was. But that's what note pads are for.

Parents, it doesn't make it any easier, but what you feel, we all feel. When my daughter gets 'down' I remind her —and me—of the motorcycle racers' motto, "when in doubt, gas it. You've got to go for it."

Her Love Still Abides:

Harry's Story

Harry lives in New York City, where he is a publisher and writer. He also enjoys hiking, painting and gardening. His wife was originally diagnosed with a low grade astrocytoma. She currently resides in a nursing home in Brooklyn. Harry has cared for his wife for over twenty years.

"Last Ode"

The day they told me you were dying, the air was
        oversexed with Spring,
the first full musky heat of Spring, and lovers
        bloomed in every park
like lilacs, and lilacs sang like love, and the song of
        lilacs smote me,
cut me open to the quick of love; lay open all the
        years onto
such a day in a little park with lilacs: God! you
        reeked of lilacs,
after having bathed in a tub of lilac water for the
        Spring, for me!
And I sneezed and laughed and gave you lilacs.

The day they told me you were dying, Death's soft
        lilac shadow bathed you
from our first Spring, renewing love, and it was the
        first Spring heat of love,

Navigating Through a Strange Land

filling us with each other, dispelling all the business
       of the years,
returning us to full-time lover, and we called our
       destiny a gift.
Finding in Death's infinite transparency all pleasures
       godly pure,
we called it lucky to be young for Death.

When you were missing from your place, I searched
       for you in the labyrinth
deep in the hospital underground. And I was
       Orpheus. *Love has led me here*
to these realms of silence and cold creation. The lords
       of those terrible abodes
trembled at my sacred rage and let me pass, hearing
       Orpheus ask,
"Where is my wife? What have you done with my wife? I
       have come for my wife.
Which wheel can spin the thread that was her life?"

When they returned you to your place, yet missing from
       yourself, pale, blighted
shadow, Death's grip graven on your brow, I learned
       to envy Orpheus.
O lucky, lucky Orpheus! For love plucked in the full
       of beauty,
for the starry lyre of lament and the consummation of
       death.
What if his Eurydice had followed from shadow into
       sunlight
yet stayed a shade *forever lost* beside him, without a
       last farewell.
I make a lyre of lilacs for my wife.

                        —Harry

(originally published in Two Friends II, 1988; Harry Smith and Menke
Katz, Birch Brook Press, 1988, pages 81-82)

Family Members Tell Their Stories

I liken the loss of my wife to the Orpheus legend, except that I envy Orpheus for losing his wife completely while everything was still beautiful. My Eurydice is in a nursing home several blocks away, alive but forever lost, like a ghost. She can not talk, nor learn anything new, nor walk, and seems to have little awareness of her situation. I believe that she recognizes me and our children and a few old friends. She is somewhat responsive and can communicate pleasure or displeasure and affection through facial expressions. She is paralyzed on one side; she gestures with her good hand occasionally, usually to indicate irritation. She can also hold hands and reciprocate a kiss. The ability to love seems to abide after most of the other mental abilities are gone.

It is now about seventeen years since she was diagnosed as having a left frontal astrocytoma classified as moderate. Being alive, she is a statistical success, as nearly all the people with the same affliction would have died within the first five years and the majority within three years. She is a private patient at the nursing home and has a private companion who feeds and nurses her. She is in no pain, except when she aspirates. Because eating, even the mush that she must be given, is one of her few pleasures, I have not authorized the insertion of a feeding tube. Her impairment is caused by injured and dead brain cells all across the frontal region, a product of high-level radiation therapy.

Ironically, she had frequently asked about the possibility of impairment from the treatment, and at every step we had been reassured that it was not a possibility to be feared, that the main danger was the progress of the tumor itself, which was effectively "sterilized." There is continuing necrosis of the brain cells, thus the possibility of more strokes (she had one three years after the radiation) and arterial occlusions. Had she known what would befall her, she never would have consented to the treatment.

In 1977, she was operated on by a neurosurgeon at a University Hospital, who removed the ventricular blockage, as best he could. Another doctor then administered the radiation. A couple of weeks after in-hospital radiation therapy, the residual mass swelled, causing blockage again. She was in pain so severe that she was unable to move from a fetal position. The neurosurgeon operated again to install a shunt. She developed severe aphasis during the radiation treatment, which mostly disappeared several weeks later. Her hospitalization for the treatment lasted more than two months.

Previously, for the diagnosis, she had been hospitalized for three weeks by a neurologist. Some kind of glioma had been suspected, but the species of tumor was not determined until after the operation.

Probably she had been affected by it for a least a year, possibly two years, before the diagnosis. She had lacked most of the classic symptoms of a brain tumor—dropping things, stumbling, radical behavior changes. Looking back, I'm quite sure that she had stumbled a few times while hurrying, which I'd considered unusual because she was a graceful person, and her walking had slowed. She always had suffered from frequent headaches, but they gradually had become worse and more frequent. One internist had treated her for sinusitis; then an ear, nose and throat physician treated her for neuralgia. Only after her symptoms had escalated to include episodes of projectile vomiting, temporary blindness and diplopia (double vision) did another doctor send her to a neurologist.

Before that, she'd considered going to a psychiatrist because she'd felt increasingly unable to cope with our children and the household and her career opportunities. She had recently gone back to school, obtaining an M.A. in psychology and had a few courses toward a Ph.D. Then she stopped her studies and neglected to pursue a job which she had wanted.

In the few weeks between her diagnosis and her treatment (while waiting to see what the lesion would look like in a second CT-scan, a month after the first), we had some of the best times of our lives.

After the treatment, there were about three years when she was outwardly normal, able to walk and talk, even score well on an intelligence test. Yet she was very impaired. Motivation itself was impaired. She no longer had the ability to decide to go anywhere, do anything on her own, and became totally dependent on me. She paid little attention to our three teenage children, and usually was confused about what they were doing. Her ability to retain new information was very limited; thus she became very forgetful, typically unable to recall daily events. Sometimes she got lost.

Then she had a major stroke, three years later (again the result of the brain damage), at first being totally paralyzed on the left side and without speech, (after which she was hospitalized for about a month). With physical therapy she learned how to walk again with a quad cane; most of her speech came back (she had some speech therapy). She kept on that plateau for perhaps a year. A stair elevator had been installed in our brownstone, and I had hired a nursing aide, the same woman who cares for her now. A slow decline then proceeded, speech becoming less and less, confusion becoming pervasive. About seven years ago, despite anti-convulsant drugs, she suffered a seizure lasting several days, lost almost all of her speech and ability to care for herself. Subject to very frequent seizures and swallowing problems from then on, it was no longer possible to care for her at home. At that time she became a resident of the Cobble Hill Nursing Home in Brooklyn.

In the years when she was an invalid and at home, I took her for Caribbean vacations every winter in a wheelchair and to Maine in the summers. While she still enjoyed travelling in these years, despite the difficulties (for instance, I would have to ask strangers to help her in the ladies room and sometimes entered one myself if she fell), she was usually disoriented (at a resort in Jamaica, say, she might think she was on a boat) and sometimes she would manage to hobble off by herself on some imaginary errand (in the absence of memory, any vagrant thought or dream seemed real to her).

In her current condition she is serene. Like a slow child, she plays with stuffed animals; she has many plants in her room and looks at them often. Of course, she can no longer read but looks at pictures in magazines. She is apparently unaware of time, and in some ways, at the age of fifty-six, she is remarkably untouched by time— no wrinkles, only a few streaks of gray in her dark brown hair. She is free of care and well-cared for. Obviously she is an easy patient and smiles beatifically at those who are kind, so she is popular with the staff, and her regular private aide is very devoted.

I visit most days when I am in New York, but my absences become longer. Now I go to Downeast Maine in all seasons and stay for the greater part of the summer there at my country place, and I travel more on business. Another woman became my companion several years ago. Before that, when I reached the age of forty-eight, about nine years ago, the same age at which my father had died of a heart attack, I went through an intense middle-aged fool phase for a year, dating dozens of women, even several very young women who had interned with me. I offered them "ideal nights," anything they wished, any place they wanted to go.

I have not gone to any of the relatives' meetings at the nursing home, but I used to go to all such sessions when my wife was being treated at the University Hospital. Many people of course feel guilt about not having been good enough to their loved ones before, and not being good enough with them during their illness, often even resenting the sick person because of the hardships being caused. I never had those problems. Rightly or wrongly—probably wrongly, there was a persistent belief among the relatives that their loved ones over-sensitivity to the stress of life and difficulties in personal relationships actually caused the malignant tumors. These sessions, on the whole, seemed useful to me and most of the other people.

I am bitter about our experiences with the doctors, but I temper that with understanding of human fallibility. I tell myself that the average internist encounters only one or two brain tumor patients in a lifetime of practice, and their misdiagnoses probably made no difference in the long-term outcome. As to the tragic course of treatment, I have no doubt that the neurosurgeon thought he would succeed in giving her considerably more time of enjoyable life and did not foresee what would happen. After all, he was a superstar: books have been written about him. A Bogart-like personality, the hospital staff trembled when they heard that he was about to reach the floor. He was very hard on the other doctors, but he had unlimited patience in answering questions from his patients and their relatives (not always correctly, as it turned out) and, despite being the busiest neurosurgeon in town, always returned phone calls the same day.

However, when the chief resident asked him if he was going to install a ventricular shunt at the same time as he operated on the tumor, he said, "A human being is not a machine.... I think I can unblock her." That proved to be a wrong decision, but I think that he had not wished to mar her beauty. Strangely, her beauty was mentioned in the medical charts, which nurses told me was unprecedented.

Three years later, after the catastrophic stroke, he would have nothing to do with her case. I can accept that people make mistakes, or that things don't always go exactly the way you intend; but we felt shoved aside afterward, and that was the most painful of all.

I also felt that more could be done with family members who visit in the hospital. It would have helped me to have something to do during the long months of daily visits, often six hours at a time. It would have helped to be a part of the rehabilitation process and be able to constructively help her when this was still possible.

Chapter Four

Professional Caregivers

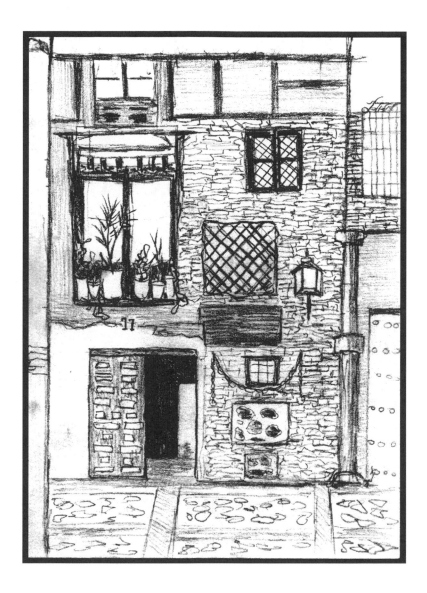

Modern Fiction on the Couch:

An Interview with a Retired

Psychoanalyst

When Anatole Broyard, former book review editor of the New York *Times*, questioned a retiring psychoanalyst on the difference between characters in fiction and his patients, he responded: "When I look back on them, it almost seems that my patients were more original—I'm tempted to say more talented—than people in many current novels."

"When someone tells me his story, he's fighting for his life, his happiness, his truth, if you like. He puts everything he has into his narrative... Such pure need poured out of the people I saw, such beautiful sadness, such a reaching for the past or future, that I couldn't help loving them... They may have felt that I alone understood them; I was the repository of their hopes and fears, their secrets. In a sense I was the mirror on the wall that enabled them to imagine for a moment that they were the fairest of them all, for there are times in analysis when nearly every patient takes on a great beauty, the beauty, you might say, of being the only creature who has to struggle with consciousness."

Yet I don't always feel this pressing toward clarification in novels. The characters don't talk with the same urgency. It's as if they haven't much faith in whomever they're performing for. Authors who aren't faithful to their characters remind me of people who lie about their dreams."

"One lets the men and women in a novel speak or act for themselves, and the situation in analysis is similar. Much of what I do is simply sit and wait while the patient shows himself to himself. Eventually, if we're lucky, something happens—something that he wants and needs and has been desperately waiting for. But in quite a few novels I read, I don't feel much wanting or needing, which baffles and frustrates me."

"One of the things that has always moved me in analysis was the patient's voice. No singer or composer could express all the changes of voice that an excited, grieving or raging human being produces. But current fiction tends to be curiously dispassionate in its voice, I don't hear the break and tide of rhythm, the pulling for breath, the squawk or shriek of certain words, like bird or animal cries. And the images—those creatures from the black lagoon that used to haunt my consultation room—where are they?"

"Then there were patients who would try to impress me with their brilliance or wit, as if to show that they didn't need me, didn't need anything. Certain authors are like that, and I want to ask them, Are you satisfied just to be amusing? What are you concealing?"

"Tell me," he said, "What you do miss most? "What did your patients give you that fiction doesn't?" He thought a while. "Incongruity," he said. "Most of all I miss incongruity. A psychoanalyst, or at least this one, is constantly refreshed—even sustained—by the gorgeous incongruities that people produce under stress. Such a wrench of perspective is a measure of our range, our suppleness. Occasionally a patient will go through the kind of abrupt self-transcendence that's one of the glories of our species. Without transition, he'll leap from the disgusting to the sublime, from the petty or mundane to the wildest shores of human sensibility. These flashes of incongruity are like dying and going to heaven. If I wrote a novel, I would fill it with incongruities like kisses."

Have you ever found any writers you envy because they came closer to the human soul than you did?" he asked.

"Oh, yes. Indeed yes. There are certainly exceptions. Once in a while a novelist will raise a question and carry it to a height too exquisite to be described in any but ontological or theological terms. He'll develop his character's difficulty to a point where it dissolves into a radiance, a beatitude. It will have all the pathos of human fallibility, of original sin. It will identify our limits, and there's a consolation in this that only a few of us have the courage to appreciate. If a patient came to me with a complaint of such grandeur, I'd send him away. I'd tell him his difficulty is worth living for, worth suffering for, even worth dying for. I know this is romantic, but that's what psychoanalysis should be: a romance, or roman, an art form."

Focus on the Things You Can Control: Charlie Wilson, M.D.

Dr. Charles Wilson is Professor and former Chairman of the Department of Neurological Surgery at the University of California, San Francisco, and Director of the Brain Tumor Research Center. He is originally from Missouri. In his spare time he enjoys running and playing jazz piano. This essay was adapted from his speech given at the National Brain Tumor Foundation's Third Biannual Conference, March 10-13, 1994, and printed with the permission of NBTF and the author.

When you or someone close to you has a diagnosis of a brain tumor, there are three immediate effects: one is practical, how will this affect your life; the second is physical, you may have some after affects from the tumor; and the third, which I will discuss, is the psychological.

There's first the event, but more importantly, there's the individual's perception of that event's effect on them and their lives, both immediately and in the future. And, it is perfectly normal at this time to have very deep emotions about such an event. They need to be acknowledged, and if they aren't acknowledged, they can prove to be very damaging. Some of the emotions we feel are helplessness, and then often hopelessness, and the two are very closely intermingled.

Secondly, you go through a period of bereavement, whether you are the patient or a member of the family. This was eloquently discussed by Dr. Elizabeth Kubler Ross in her first book *On Death and Dying*, where she described the phases of which many of you are familiar - the shock and denial, the anger and rage, the deep depression, which if prolonged can be deeply damaging, and finally acceptance. (She has another book which I would recommend to you called *Living with Death and Dying*.)

Acceptance, however, is not resignation. Resignation is what I call the white flag; you're resigned to what you've heard, or to what you even may believe. To accept that you have a brain tumor and that things may not look too good is one thing, but to resign to its inevitable fate, I think, is quite another.

Science has tried to discover the mechanisms for these powerful effects that our emotions have on our health, and this has given rise to terms such as psycho-neuro-endocrine effects and psycho-neuro-immune effects.

I'm often asked, "Does stress cause cancer?" I mean, who among us is not subjected to stress in some form. However, there is a basic hypothesis in science called the immune surveillance hypothesis, and the hypothesis is this: that every single day something we eat or breath carries in it something that may cause a cell to mutate and to become a cancer cell, but we have this healthy immune system and that particular cell is destroyed and never becomes a cancer.

It is unlikely that stress directly causes cancer, but I now think it can unmask or certainly accelerate the appearance of cancer. This comes from a hard core scientist who a few short years ago thought this was nonsense. I believe also that stress can play a role in both progression of disease and in recurrence of a tumor.

Stress can become very powerful. It is that strong emotion that leads to world class performance; but it has to be harnessed so that it can be a positive power, and not something that has an erosive consequence.

Robert Saposwki has written a book called *Why Zebras Don't Get Ulcers*. What he points out is that stress is very essential for us to react to a number of things in our lives. But, an appropriate five minute response to stress becomes very destructive when that five minutes becomes five days, five weeks, and five months.

The highest court of science in this country is the National Institutes of Health. They have established, in the past two years, an office of alternative medicine. In part it's to investigate scientific claims, such as for Leatrile. But, it's also acknowledging that there are nonscientific factors that have to do with disease and health and survival.

In January of this year the National Cancer Institute (NCI) put on a symposium, and the title was Mind/Body

Interaction in Disease. Bernie Siegel introduced the mind/body connection. Then there was the very popular Bill Moyers book and PBS special Healing and the Mind.

One, from this, could conclude that the mind is powerful, that this power can be developed, and directed positively.

Who has not heard of spontaneous remission and spontaneous regression of cancer. It's been documented many times over, particularly in tumors of a limited sort: neuroblastomas, malignant melanomas, and lymphomas. Sometimes there is an explanation, an infection for example. It's been known that if you had cancer of the lung and developed a complication, that is, a cancer in the plural cavity where the tumor was removed, that your chances of survival were very much better. And it has also been shown for a glioblastoma that if you got a post surgical infection it was statistically significant.

And there are other reasons we can sometimes point to as the basis for spontaneous remission; pregnancy, partial removal of the tumor; fever from a non infectious sort. Often the basis for this is the immune system, but often we simply do not know why.

I will leave you with ten very specific things that you can do, not instead of conventional medicine, but in addition to. And the point of this is that there are certain things you can't control: you can't control that you have the tumor; you can't control where it is. But there are things you can control. So, rather than be dismayed and depressed over those things you can't control, you focus on things over which you do have some control. And I can assure you that in these things that I'll recommend there is real power.

First , seek psychological help. On the front page of today's San Francisco Examiner is Mind and Matter, a story of sports psychology. These are world class athletes who often scoffed at the idea of needing any kind of psychological help. But you'd have to be pretty out of it not to recognize that sports psychology is a big thing. The Oakland A's have a full time sports psychologist on staff.

So there has to be a power within psychologically examining ourselves—who we are, our strengths, our weaknesses—that helps us in dealing with our lives and whatever life may bring us. But I think more importantly, from your standpoint, empowering you in a way that has been shown many times to increase your chance of survival and have a profound effect of longevity. By this I mean learning coping skills, and how to manage stress, whether this is by meditation, or by some breathing exercise, but something that you can be taught to do that gives you some sense of having control over what's happening.

Second, socialize, socialize, socialize, with your friends, with your family. Dr. Spiegel's work with breast cancer patients showed that those who became socially isolated had a mortality rate twice as high as those who were not socially isolated; a very impressive statistic. If a patient has at least one confidant, a person to whom they can tell everything, their chances of surviving over any given period of time is approximately doubled. There are those who say a pet has the same effect.

Third, join a support group. Someplace where you can go and express your frights, your worries, your concerns, where you can laugh and you can bond with people who happen to end up in the same boat you find yourself in.

Four, learn about your disease. Initially it's very stressful. You read about brain tumors, you see what a scan looks like; you see own scan. You get tight in the throat, almost sick in the stomach. But once you have learned something about your disease, you become a partner in the team of people who will determine your future treatment. And, over time, this improves your ability to cope. It's simply that, instead of a black box, it's something you at least have some understanding of.

Five, grieve. It's a terrible thing that has happened. Your family grieves, you grieve, and it's OK, it's natural.

Six, face your own mortality. This was the hardest one for me. As I whiz by my 60th birthday, and I'm looking forward, in a couple of months, to my 65th, I am in touch, finally, with my own mortality. I've always been too busy to think about it! I realize that life is finite, life can be beautiful, but it's certainly not forever. A part of the end of life is dying and it's OK to think about it. It's OK to wonder about it. It's OK to be a little bit afraid of it. But, it's not OK to just pretend it will never happen to you.

Seven, try to learn something about visual imaging, and there's many ways of doing that. Dr. Martin Rossman, of San Francisco, has introduced interactive guided imagery, which is just one form. I used to think this was not very important. But I'm now persuaded that for some people—maybe not for you, certainly not for all—it can be very powerful.

Eight, despite all that has happened, decide that you are going to develop some new interest, or some new activity. Maybe you've always wanted to go down to a church and become a volunteer. Maybe you've always said you'd like to take a class in Greek mythology. Maybe you'd like to learn jazz sax, write a book, learn to paint. Doing something that's different is compelling and will give you a sense of new accomplishment.

Nine, exercise and eat properly. You say, "Well I have a weak leg or arm," or "I'm on Decadron, and I don't have much energy." Well, if you want to be inspired, just look in some day on the Special Olympics, or watch a wheelchair marathon. Exercise gives you a sense of discipline, a sense of control, it makes you feel better. Psychiatrists learned long ago that probably exercise is more effective for depression than the couch.

Eat properly. You should be healthy. Just because you have a brain tumor, does not mean that the body that happens to be harboring this tumor should be allowed to go along without maintenance, and improve it. If you think vitamins will help, vitamins will help.

Finally, get in touch with some higher being, and it can be many forms, many spirits. It will give you a strength, it will give you a peace. Physicians are now learning that when religion matters to a patient, they should take that seriously. The mind can be a powerful determinant in healing and recovery. Believe that you can beat this disease against all odds. Focus on those things in your life that you can control, but above all, put your trust in a higher spirit, because the strength that you can find in a spiritual experience has power beyond your imagination.

It's a beautiful day today. It's the first day of the rest of your life, and I hope that my God, and your God, will bless you all.

Every Tumor Has a Brain—

Assessing Neurological Change:

John Walker, Ph.D.

John is Assistant Professor of Neuropsychology, in the Department of Neurology, and Director of the Northern California Epilepsy Center at the University of California, San Francisco, and has worked with many brain tumor patients. He is originally from Wisconsin, and now makes his home in San Rafael, California.

"The human brain is a world consisting of a number of explored continents and great stretches of unknown territory"

—Ramon y Cajal

I have worked with a number of people with brain injuries in my career as a neuropsychologist. In each case I have tried to bring my knowledge of brain sciences, and my knowledge of human thinking and emotion, to help both the person and me to understand what has occurred. Each person is unique, not only in such medical factors as the location, size and type of tumor, but also in how it has affected that person's functions, and how the person has responded to the illness.

Although I feel that each person is unique, there are some patterns that emerge across individuals. I want to share with you a review of those patterns, to guide you in evaluating whether you are relatively typical, or relatively atypical of some known patterns that occur in people with brain tumors.

I'll mostly focus on the things I know best, which are human cognition, or thinking, as well as emotion. Each person who comes to me with a brain tumor has two things that I consider: First, I want to know something about the location, size, and type of tumor, as well as where the person is in their treatment. Second, I want to know how the tumor has affected the person. I want to know whether there have been changes in perception, motor abilities, language, memory, and other aspects of thinking. I also want to know how the person is coping with their illness.

I'm aware that for the person with the tumor, the problems may be new, and confusing. I feel my job is to try to help make some sense out of the symptoms. Usually this evaluation helps someone who is a long-term survivor of a brain tumor. Sometimes the effort is directed toward helping a person and family understand the changes that are happening as the tumor progresses. Both situations have value.

I use several guiding principles. First, I listen carefully to what the person, or their family, have noticed so far. I want to get a good sense of what they feel is the pattern of strengths and weaknesses, what has been changed and what is unchanged. I know that I will meet with the person for only a short time, and many real-life problems may not be apparent in an office examination.

Second, I follow a rule, which I call Walker's Law, which says "The customer is always right", and so I want to be clear about what the person or family think are the problems. However, there's another part of Walker's Law, which says "The customer may be right, but for the wrong reason." That is, often people notice a problem, but may have the wrong explanation.

One of my favorite examples is a woman named Eileen who came to see me because she felt she had a bad memory. She told me that when people came up to her, saying hello, she would have no idea who the person was until there was enough said to finally trigger a memory. She found it very embarrassing not to recognize familiar faces. Eileen had a brain tumor removed as a teen, almost 20 years before I met her. She had also had complications of hydrocephalus.

In examining Eileen I discovered that she was nearly blind, which she readily acknowledged. She had even been to the School for the Blind for rehab. She could see nothing from her right eye. Her left eye allowed a small field of vision, about like that you'd have looking through the cardboard tube from paper towels. Within that field of vision she usually ignored the left half of the image, favoring the right half of her visual world. Yet the nature of her brain injury had been to make her feel that her vision was perfectly intact, except when someone called it to her attention. It wasn't surprising that she didn't recognize friends' faces—she got very little visual input, and it was only when they spoke long enough that she could place them. But her problem in this situation was due to vision, not memory.

The example I gave above also illustrates the third part of my approach to understanding a person's brain function, called the "Principle of Parsimony." This is a concept in science that says we favor simpler explanations over more complex explanations. Since vision is a simpler, earlier stage of information processing than memory, if vision is impaired that will explain an apparent memory problem better than expecting that memory itself is impaired. I feel it's important to understand what is causing an impairment, as the first step toward overcoming that impairment. Often understanding that the problem exists at a simpler level of information processing offers clues for how to work around the problem.

When considering the functional effects of a brain tumor, several biological characteristics help to narrow the possibilities. First, for most functions the left side of the brain controls the right side of the body, and vice-versa. This applies to important functions such as skin sensation and motor control.

Professional Caregivers

Other senses, such as vision and hearing, are more complicated because there is partial crossover from the primary sense. For example, the left side of the brain monitors the right side of the visual world, taking inputs from each eye. A person with a tumor affecting visual centers in the brain, for example, may make a person insensitive to one side of the visual world, even though each eye remains capable of vision. Tumors that affect visual pathways may selectively knock out only parts of the visual world, which in fact is used by the doctors as an important clue for where a tumor might be located.

Another strong biological predictor comes from observations that most people have their ability to speak only in the left side of the brain. If a person has a tumor in the left, this is far more likely to cause some degree of language problem than the same tumor in the right side. However, about 10% of people have their speech mostly on the right side. This appears to be more likely if a person is left-handed, though most left-handers still have speech on the left side of the brain. Because speech is such an important function for humans, problems are often obvious.

Depending on the location of the tumor a person may have mostly problems speaking, or mostly problems understanding, or may have more limited problems such as difficulty repeating back something, or difficulty with reading, or writing, or spelling. Almost all people with language impairment will have problems with word-finding, that is, an extreme version of the tip-of-the-tongue phenomenon everybody experiences. A thorough evaluation of language strengths and weaknesses can be very helpful in these situations.

Once we get past such elementary functions as vision, hearing, skin sensation, motor control and language, we are hard-pressed to locate functions in particular spots in the brain. Studies of patients with brain tumors, as well as people with other kinds of brain injuries, suggest that some functions may be represented in both sides of the brain, with perhaps more function in one side. For example, the right side of the brain probably has greater representation for visual-spatial analysis.

The back half of the brain is primarily involved in high-level perceptual analysis, while the front part of the brain is primarily involved in evaluating and executing actions. Pathways in the temporal lobes appear to be critical to taking in and storing new information, though they appear to be unimportant in retrieving that information once it has been learned. Previously learned information appears to be stored in multiple areas of the brain, so that declines in overall "intelligence" are more closely tied to total size of injury rather than location.

In addition, a person may have problems in thinking or emotional control because of distant effects of a brain tumor or its consequences. For example, brain tumors grow and occupy space within a limited area, inside the skull. This growth can lead to pressure effects on the brain, especially reflected in problems with concentration or even level of arousal. A person may feel more irritable, or emotionally out of control. Some tumors affect the circulation of fluid inside the brain, which can lead to a buildup of fluid (hydrocephalus), which can lead to increased pressure, with effects similar to those described above.

Some tumors, especially those affecting "white matter," which are the connecting fibers in the brain, may block effective transmission from one brain area to another even though the primary brain areas are intact. Sometimes the treatments for brain tumors lead to temporary, diffuse problems with thinking skills, especially seen in chemotherapy or radiation sickness. Sometimes in an effort to stop the tumor healthy brain cells are permanently damaged, often in the area nearby the tumor, but sometimes in more distant places.

Many people with brain tumors can benefit from a systematic evaluation of their intellectual strengths and weaknesses. There are hundreds, if not thousands of tests that have been developed to test brain function. In general a good neuropsychological evaluation should cover a variety of the abilities that might be affected by a brain tumor. This would include, at a minimum, an evaluation of verbal and visual skills, as well as verbal and visual memory, in addition to tests of concentration, motor speed and control. The total time devoted to such testing may vary from less than an hour to many hours, and should reflect the nature of the problem and the needs for assistance. Sometimes subtle problems require more evaluation than obvious problems.

I think a good evaluation should also be tied to real-world concerns. The same deficit may affect two individual's lives in very different ways. A salesman who develops language problems will be affected very differently than a gardener, though both may have problems. Similarly, two persons with visual-spatial problems will be affected differently if one is a plumber and the other a clerical worker. It is not enough to define how a person did on a series of tests—there should be relevance to that person's real-world needs.

Finally, the person with a brain tumor does not exist in an emotional vacuum. Although some types of brain injury can directly affect emotional state, most usually the emotions shown by a person with a brain tumor reflect that persons' reaction to the situation. In particular, if the effects of the tumor have been to impair an ability that person felt was essential, depression will commonly occur. In addition, it is common for a person to go through various phases, ranging from anxiety about the future, depression about losses, or to exhilaration at being alive, and determination to live as fully as possible.

They don't necessarily occur in the same order for each person. For most people this may even change from day to day, depending on the stage of the illness. It is important to understand that anxiety and depression may in themselves decrease cognitive function, and effective treatment may dramatically restore cognitive function.

I must say I always admire those individuals who are stubborn, and won't let the tumor stop them. I think the best most of us can strive for is to develop a sense of realistic hopefulness, based on acceptance of what has occurred, and a positive attitude to strive for improvement in the future. The basis for that hopefulness should be a clear understanding of what is and is not possible concerning improved brain function.

Finally, I want to say a few words about how to search out someone who can help determine how the brain is functioning, and how it might be improved. Usually the doctors most involved in a person with a brain tumor are the neurosurgeons and neurooncologists. Although some are very knowledgeable about how the brain functions, most do not have an extensive background in cognition or emotional evaluation. Other doctors, such as neurologists or psychiatrists often are more knowledgeable about such things, and neuroscience nurses often have a great deal of hands-on experience.

Psychologists, especially neuropsychologists, are usually very well-equipped to evaluate the cognitive and emotional consequences of a brain tumor, but other specialists, such as speech therapists, occupational therapists, and physical therapists have a great deal to offer, too, depending on a person's specific needs.

Navigating Through a Strange Land

Most importantly, I think, is finding that professional who has a knack for assessing not only performance in the office, but how that translates to the real world, and what rehabilitation is available based on the outcome of the tests. It's fair to push any of your doctors though for as much information as you can get, and to ask them to refer you to the other specialists listed above. You, and your family, are the ones who live every day with the consequences of the brain tumor, and you deserve the best insight possible about your brain's function.

Dedicated to Stacy

What About Our Faith?—Reflections of a Hospital Chaplain: Karyn's Story

In 1988, Karyn wrote a story for Search, NBTF's newsletter, when I was editor about her husband, Bruce Shadbolt, who was struggling with his brain tumor. They lived in Hawaii at the time. Bruce eventually died, and Karyn moved to California, studied theology, and recently remarried. She is now Director of Pastoral Care at Long Beach Memorial Medical Center, in Long Beach, California.

Let me introduce my family, a family of performers, a family of achievers. We helped others, they came to us for advice. We were self-sufficient. We didn't need anyone. We were good at all we did. Bruce ran a successful company, played semipro soccer, coached and sang the tenor leads in major operas and oratorios. I ran an advertising agency, and sang lead roles in musicals, operas and oratorios. Jim was the drum major and a radio disk jockey at 17, Debbie was outstanding thespian as a freshman, winning many statewide talent and beauty contests. At four, Matthew was already playing soccer and winning baby contests. Our family sang together professionally. We thought there was nothing that we couldn't handle, and handle well. We were active in church, but, it was like a second job. We believed that we were touched by God with special blessing.

There were challenges though. My adopted Mom, a few close friends called her Tutu, was dying of cancer. I had been caring for her for several years. Her illness had overlapped that of her husband. He had died in 1983 after suffering five heart attacks and three strokes. Tutu was now near death in Queens Hospital. I was managing to work full time, keep house, take care of the kids and be with her in the hospital each day, all without asking for any help. God was blessing me with strength. I was proud of my performance.

During that year, my husband Bruce had been acting strangely. He was a perfectionist, but things were not always getting done. He had started to sleep instead of doing chores. He was known for his calm personality, a thinker that didn't give in to much emotion. He never raised his voice. He now yelled at the kids, even using profanity. His customers complained of inefficiency. I thought our marriage was on the rocks. I believed he was working too hard in his business, and just didn't have enough left over for us. I looked for psychological reasons for the changes... considered divorce.

Bruce was a pillar of the church. He often preached and taught. He was a Bible scholar. After church one

Professional Caregivers

Sunday, a friend came to talk with me. "Something happened to Bruce when we were together, maybe a seizure." He knew that my "mom" was dying and didn't want to add to my grief, but felt he needed to let me know.

That night, in the dark, I confronted Bruce with the information. He cried, and admitted that for several months his mind had not been doing what he wanted it to. When he wanted the window down in the car, he reached for the radio. He couldn't always turn off the shower. He was having spells where he would just lose awareness. He would still be awake and standing, but not functioning. He could tell when the "spells" were coming and warn people not to be alarmed.. just to wait them out. Later, clients and our young son told of times when he was driving, when he would just continue into intersections, or stop in the midst of traffic. He hadn't wanted to bother me when I had my plate full—hadn't really wanted to face the fact that something serious was going on. We prayed together that God would take away our fear.

After three appointments with the neurologist, a CAT scan was ordered. He was diagnosed with a glioblastoma multiforme, grade IV. His prognosis was 2-6 months. The day after his first surgery at Queens Hospital, my "mom" died on the 7th floor. I planned her funeral outside of the intensive care unit. I wanted so much just to sit and tell her all of this. How could this be happening to us? We did everything right. We were good Christians. We helped others. We read our Bible.

Navigating Through a Strange Land

We began to get advice. I had been the soloist for the Christian Science church for nine years. They came to make a pastoral call. They said that there was no intelligence in matter, and that all was mind. They asked us to change our thinking, not to give in to the information that we had been given. They asked us to believe that God only gave perfection to God's children, all we had to do was believe it. We tried...

Our daughter had joined a charismatic church. She and her boyfriend and their pastor came to call. They told us that it was simple, if you only had "enough faith" the brain tumor would be healed. We prayed and asked for enough faith. It was hard to imagine just exactly what that would be. We wondered who was measuring and how we would know.

Our church family came to the hospital before the first surgery. They gathered around the bed for prayer and celebrated communion. It was a wonderful feeling being surrounded by our community of faith. We felt God's presence and power. We believed that God was hearing us and would answer our prayers. There was so much more that we wanted to do. With all of this faith, surely he would have a complete physical healing.

But, passively praying wasn't enough, so after the initial shock, we jumped into our "doing" roles. We gathered information. I went to the medical library and looked up everything I could about this tumor. It wasn't going to get us down. Ten days after his initial surgery, we opened as Captain von Trapp and Maria in the Sound of Music. We attended a Marriage Encounter weekend, and sang the Hawaiian Wedding Song to the other couples, who were all in tears.

Bruce began radiation. After the six week course, the tumor had all but disappeared. We were on track, all of the prayers were being answered. Then the chemo. He did better than most, as we had expected. He was proud of his discipline. We were interviewed by the paper. We spoke to any group who would listen about how we were living with his disease. We made radio and TV appearances. We spoke at Bruce's alma mater. We spoke about faith and determination. Years later our older children told us how phoney this all seemed to them, when they were so afraid. But fear was not part of our game plan.

Then the scan following the first month of chemo. The tumor was larger than it had been originally! What about all the prayers? People said we didn't have enough faith. Once again we asked, "What was enough faith"? What about all the good we were doing for the community, our righteous and Christ-centered behavior? What about his healthy diet and visualization? What was happening? Why now... we were doing everything right? We were ashamed of the fear we felt in our hearts, too afraid to verbalize it to each other or to other "church" people. We suspected now that we didn't have "enough faith." God knew the truth, others didn't. Individually, we thought about all the unworthy things we had done and were ashamed.

Then the chance to be part of research. Off to San Francisco from our Hawaiian island home for a radioactive implant. Bruce was a scientist. He was excited about being part of such a project. They said they would blow the tumor away. We canceled our first ever family vacation and sent the kids east for Christmas. We visited the labs. He even talked about working there after he was cured. He went through the procedure with flying colors, as we would have expected. We were back on track; we had just been tested.

We left the hospital on Christmas Eve, to fly east, visit his relatives and join our children. Daily he got weaker. Finally, I could hardly wake him. He was seizing. We flew back to San Francisco and he lost consciousness. He didn't know me. This wasn't in the plan. What was going wrong? What were we to do? Where was God? Was God listening? I remembered the Psalms where the Isrealite people cried out to a God who they thought didn't hear.

What we were forced "to do" was just "to be." We had no other choice. Our minds could not solve this, medicine did not have all the answers. We were no longer wanting to "go public." After all, who wants to hear someone who is not winning. We had so much to learn. We quit being directive with God. We waited. After he regained consciousness, he was paralyzed on his left side. We flew back to Hawaii in a more introspective place.

On the plane, I promised God that since God had spared Bruce, I wanted to do something to help other patients. Soon after our arrival we started a group called "Cansurmount," with the help of the American Cancer Society. Cansurmount brought together brain tumor families and patients. As God would have it, working with these families gave us more than we gave them. Phone calls began to come from all over the world. We were not alone in our struggle. We were beginning to recognize just how important it was to have someone to share with who understood, really understood.

I had also been a perfectionist. A dinner party required at least a days work with nothing left to chance. Now our house was always filled with people. You never knew how many would be eating. The table would be littered with cardboard containers, catsup bottles, paper napkins, soda cans and smiling people. We began to learn that when you present yourself "in control," and "in charge," people are not inclined to move towards you in relationship. When everything has to be just the way you like it, some important things get lost. We began to experience what real friendship was; relationship with our friends and with God. I remember thinking that I was always praying, not in the traditional sense, but that God was always part of my thought process, walking alongside.

Navigating Through a Strange Land

The people in our church became part of our family. The other brain tumor families became our family. The house was no longer perfectly cleaned, but it was often filled with people who cared. We saw God in their faces and deeds. They cleaned, washed, cooked, shopped, (years after Bruce died, I was still hunting for things).

Through the support of our pastor, I began to read books on scripture, theology, spirituality, and psychology. Factoring our experience into these subjects expanded my understandings. I began to see what is meant by the paradoxes in the New Testament; to lose your life is to gain it... pick up your cross and follow me. I was humbled into handing my problems over to God, now that I couldn't fix them myself... be anxious for nothing, but in prayer and supplication let your requests be known to God... the world is groaning in labor pains waiting for the redemption of our bodies... The scriptures began to make sense. It was time to listen to God, instead of trying to manipulate Him.

Bruce's brain tumor journey lasted over five years. During that time, he had four brain surgeries and one back surgery. Our family structure had eroded. No one was doing their "prescribed" roles anymore. We were all different. Our young son needed hospitalization for emotional support. We were all in therapy at one time or another. The relationship with Bruce's parents became strained as we competed for his last months.

Professional Caregivers

Bruce did not have a realistic opinion of what he could and couldn't do. It was hard to allow him to be self-sufficient and watch him behind a door in case he would fall or be frustrated. Our church family and the other Cansurmount families were a help. It was important to Bruce to do as much as he could. His assistant soccer coach would park his wheelchair on the sidelines. Even though Bruce couldn't see, he would ask him for input on each of the plays. Friends at church would come and help him prepare church school lessons. When he would ramble, they would get him back on track, always with sensitivity to his feelings. I myself was not always as sensitive as I would have liked to be. I tried not to get angry. In the attempt, I shut down emotionally. I was in "survival mode." It was so painful to lose my husband, bit by bit. Now, I was a nurse. I remember early in his disease being sorry that I now had to take out the garbage, the man's job. Eventually, there was nothing that I could ask him to do.

But God was working in ways that I hadn't noticed. I had never been very sure of myself. Now, I was managing chronic crisis. I learned I could do more than I had ever imagined. I also learned that help was always there. I kept a list by the phone of people who would help me in various ways. God was embodied in the hands and feet of our friends. Bruce was sometimes unreasonable. At those times, there were neighbors who would take Matt, our youngest son, in for awhile, no questions asked.

Navigating Through a Strange Land

There were firemen I could call if he fell, and I couldn't get him up. There were other wives going through the same thing that I could call when it just seemed like too much.

Bruce died in 1989, paralyzed and blind. It had been progressive. He died at home, as he had requested, with the help of our church family and wives whose husband had already died of the same disease. It took four of us to get him bathed, dressed and into his favorite chair. Together, we were even able to carry him into a floating chair in the pool where he could rest in the Hawaiian sun. He had quite a tan on his bald head. A Morphine pack controlled the pain.

During the last two years of his illness, I was able to begin my Masters in Pastoral studies and be licensed to minister. I started an internship as a chaplain, part-time, in the same hospital where his first surgery had taken place. I quickly knew that this was where God was calling me.

With help from our church and other families and Bruce's parents, I was able to finish my degree the year after he died. I was ordained as a minister in the Christian Church, (Disciples of Christ). My son Matthew and I moved to Loma Linda where I continued my training. Currently, I serve as Director of Pastoral Care at Long Beach Memorial Medical Center. Along with caring for patients, families, and staff, I teach ministerial students how their pain and weakness can be their strength.

Professional Caregivers

I would never had wished for this to have happened in any of our lives. But life will never be the same for any of us who traveled that journey together. We learned that real relationship comes from being willing to share your life. Not just your accomplishments. Real sharing asks for vulnerability. We are not known for what we do, but for who we are. Who we are does not depend on our IQ, our prestigious position, our elaborate home, or our over-achieving children.

We are God's perfect children. In God's hands, we are perfect in our woundedness. Remember Jacob with the wound in his side. Remember Paul, blinded on the road to Damascus. They were not prepared for ministry in a Ph.D. program, they were prepared in the "school of hard knocks." God's grace fills an empty cup, not a full one. It can not be earned or manipulated. It is when we are willing to be present to God and to others in our emptiness, that we will be filled. In covenant relationship with God, there is the power to make new. What is promised in this covenant is not equilibrium, but faithfulness.

Remember these words, from old testament scholar Walter Brueggemann, "the upshot of faithfulness is not certitude, but precariousness—precariousness which requires a full repertoire of hoping, listening, and answering to life joyously. The Bible is realistic in knowing that life does not consist in pleasant growth to well-being, but it consists in painful wrenchings and surprising gifts. And over none of them do we preside."

Navigating Through a Strange Land

A Zen Approach:
Debra Jan Bibel, Ph.D.

Debra Jan is author of "Freeing the Goose in the Bottle: Discovering Zen through Science, Understanding Science through Zen."

Korean Zen master Seung Sahn visited our Zen center one evening, and offered to answer any questions about Buddhist teachings and practice. In the large audience of monks, students, and the simply curious, one man asked the Master, "I have a friend who is dying of a brain tumor. What teachings can I give him?" Without a moments hesitation, the master replied, "First do not mention death or dying. Have your friend practice breathing in and out. With each inhalation, have him concentrate on the energy and clarity of mind; with each exhalation, let him feel the expulsion of poisons. After your friend does this practice for a while, tell him that his body has a tumor, but that his true self does not die. His true self also does not live. Ask him to find his true self with each breath in and out."

Hope (Generic)

William Buchholz, M.D.

William M. Buchholz, who wrote this piece for the Journal of the American Medical Association, *is a physician in Northern California. The style is a humorous takeoff on the information written by drug companies about their drugs.*

Description
"HOPE is what gets us out of bed in the morning."

Clinical pharmacology

HOPE is a naturally occurring substance created by an individual's ability to project himself or herself into the future and imagine something better than what exists in the present. It serves as a cofactor for most purposeful behavior and is necessary for coping with fluctuating feelings of despair, depression, fear, anxiety, and uncertainty.

HOPE has three components: the individual hoping; the projection into the future (expectation); and the object, event, or state desired.

Individuals experiencing HOPE vary with respect to

the density and binding constants of HOPE receptors. There is both up-regulation and down-regulation of receptors depending on the danger of the circumstances, the individual's sense of vulnerability, and the support system available. Certain individuals have a pathological need for HOPE and are susceptible to False HOPE.

Expectation, comprising the subunits Credibility and Attainability, is conveniently measured as a vector having units of distance and difficulty. Even if there is a strong belief that a goal is possible (Credibility), if the individual perceives it to be too difficult to attain, or that it is impossible to project himself or herself into the future, Expectation will be low. Both intellectual and emotional Expectancies must be above threshold levels for HOPE to be effective.

The Object Desired is the most visible aspect of HOPE and may be expressed concretely or implied (e.g., "I hope the surgery will cure the cancer" or "I hope everything turns out all right"). The strength of HOPE often depends on the meaning or importance (Preciousness) of the Object.

Pharmacokinetics

After administration either verbally or visually, HOPE enters cortical and thalamic pathways, where it is processed for Credibility and Attainability. If receptors are blocked by depression, anxiety, or distraction, there is no binding and HOPE dissipates immediately. Depending on the number and avidity of open receptors, there is an immediate effect that has a half-life of minutes to hours. Longer effects require repeated administration. Both sensitivity and tachyphylaxis can develop depending on how often the Desired Event occurs or does not occur.

Indications

HOPE is indicated in the treatment of HOPE Deficiency, Depression, and Anxiety and to increase Motivation and Compliance with treatment. It is useful in relieving fear, pessimism, and a sense of vulnerability. It increases energy and courage in all individuals, resulting in greater likelihood of difficult goals being accomplished.

HOPE should be given at the initial diagnosis of a potentially fatal disease, at any recurrence, and when the disease is terminal. It should also be used when dealing with chronic "benign" diseases such as arthritis, diabetes, and hypertension. It should be given whenever despair is anticipated.

HOPE Deficiency (Hopelessness) is a state of despair characterized by inability to anticipate any positive outcome. Patients are generally unable to act decisively, make decision, have meaningful relationships, or experience joy or meaning. They are described as having "given up." The Will to Live is diminished in proportion to the degree of hopelessness.

Navigating Through a Strange Land

Contraindications
There are no known contraindications for giving HOPE.

Mechanisms of Action
Depression is characterized by the inability to imagine anything different from the present. HOPE, because of the component of Expectation, relieves the inability to project into the future. HOPE allows such individuals to create a possible future, thereby relieving the onus of living in the present. The anticipation of pleasure relieves pessimism. Anxiety, characterized by a sense of loss of control, is alleviated by predicting a desirable future event, thereby providing an anchor for the individual in the midst of free-floating anxiety. The sense of aloneness is relieved by anticipating allies or help. Fear, which consists of projecting into the future an undesirable event (helplessness, pain, etc.) is redirected by the expectancy of a positive rather than negative outcome. Motivation to accomplish goals and compliance with medical treatment are increased by a sense that the goal is attainable.

Warnings
False HOPE is the intentional in inadvertent creation of the expectancy that a low-probability outcome is likely. It is a violation of medical ethics to deceive a patient intentionally for the purposes of manipulating his or her

behavior. Physicians and nurses generally try to avoid any appearance of False HOPE and may generate False Despair instead. Certain individuals, because of a high need for HOPE based on the seriousness of their condition or their premorbid personality characteristics, are prone to misinterpret information given and develop False HOPE or False Despair even then none is intended. Patients generally use False HOPE to diminish the full emotional impact of an intolerable situation.

False Despair is the intentional or inadvertent discrediting of any probability that a desired outcome is possible. To avoid any suggestion of False Hope, some medical professionals will purposely lower patient expectations to avoid any chance of disappointment. Patients likewise may avoid the disappointment of unrealized hopes by purposefully keeping the expectations low, feeling it is safer to expect the worst. It is a violation of compassion and the Hippocratic oath purposely to withhold HOPE of a low but finite probability outcome from those patients who desire it. It may be pointed out that even under the bleakest of circumstances there are some survivors.

Usage in Pregnancy and Children

HOPE is safe during Pregnancy. It passes into the breast milk and is known to be safe for infants. HOPE may be used in the pediatric population, adjusting language but not dosage according to age.

Navigating Through a Strange Land

Adverse Reactions

Adverse reactions occur when physicians or nurses, out of a desire to please the patients, try to appear more powerful than they are and manipulate patient behavior by substituting False HOPE for True or Realistic HOPE. Patients likewise may distort ethically administered True HOPE out of an inability to cope with reality. False HOPE leads to persistent denial of reality and poor judgment. It causes 1) persistent goal oriented behavior toward an unobtainable goal, 2) distraction from necessary activities, and 3) delay in resolving emotional issues. There are no adverse effects of True HOPE.

Overdose

Individuals' capacities for HOPE vary considerably. Excess True HOPE is very rare. More common is the medical personnel's assessment that the patient's estimate of outcomes is "unrealistic." Conflict arises when the patient's need for HOPE differs from the nurse's or physician's. If overdosage is suspected, however, the patient must be assessed carefully and the consequences of acute HOPE Deficiency considered. Acute HOPE Deficiency may precipitate sudden depression and increased anxiety. Withdrawal of HOPE must be done slowly and gently.

Professional Caregivers

Withdrawal

If it is determined that the patient is using False HOPE and suffering one or more of the above-mentioned adverse reactions and the danger of continued False HOPE state is greater than precipitating Acute HOPE Deficiency, withdrawal may be undertaken carefully. Efforts should be made to substitute another goal for the previous unobtainable one, preserving the positive expectancy while the goal is shifted. This may be done more easily if it is recognized that the patient is actually in a HOPE Deficiency state of fear and depression.

Dosage and Administration

Dosage and duration of treatment must be individualized. The only limit on maximum dosage is the patient's ability to receive and the professional's ability to administer HOPE at an appropriate rate.

HOPE must be administered in a form compatible with the patient's receptor system. Patients with Factual HOPE Receptors are best given HOPE in the form of facts and statistics, phrased according to "the glass is half full" philosophy. For patients with a preponderance of Emotional HOPE Receptors who manifest symptoms of anxiety and depression, HOPE should be administered in a form that can be digested emotionally. "Living proof" stories about other patients who have done well in similar circumstances are more easily accepted and can be applied directly to emotional wounds.

Navigating Through a Strange Land

At the time of diagnosis: Because excessive Information may block receptor sites for HOPE, patients' needs should be determined before either Information or HOPE is given. Open-ended questions such as "What have you been told?" or "What do you think is the matter?" will elicit responses that indicate primary needs for Information (intellectual) or encouragement (emotional). Information should be given in amounts that will not overwhelm the patient's ability to incorporate it. Such overload increases the distortion of the Information and produces either anxiety or numbness. Unless specific actions based on the Information must be taken immediately, attending to emotional needs by giving HOPE first before Information will create a more credible physician-patient or nurse-patient relationship.

During therapy: HOPE is easily administered with technical interventions. Patient HOPE may exceed the professional's HOPE. If HOPE is necessary for the patient to cope and there is no contraindication (see False HOPE above), then HOPE should be maintained as long as possible.

When "nothing else can be done:" This is the most critical situation in which HOPE must be administered. Both medical personnel and patients must shift the object of HOPE to something that is more credibly obtainable, maintaining a positive expectancy while changing goals. Generally it is possible to offer HOPE for comfort. It is always possible to offer the commitment to be there for patients as they die. Often, that is enough.

How Supplied

There is no standard dose. Individual patient needs and individual personnel styles determine how HOPE should be given. Listening carefully to both verbal and nonverbal communication will often suggest the best preparation of HOPE to use. Sometimes it is pointing out that even though the chances are slender, there is at least a chance. Sometimes it is just being there, with a gentle smile and a promise not to abandon the patient. Sometimes the greatest challenge is keeping a sufficient supply on hand for the personnel dispensing it.

The Patient and Physician Have to Fight Together: Nicholas de Tribolet, M.D.

Dr. de Tribolet is Professor and Chairman of Neurosurgery at the Centre Hospitalier Universitaire Vaudois in Lausanne, Switzerland.

I remember very clearly the first patient I had to operate on under my own responsibility. He was 20 years old, a healthy mountaineer, and Swiss champion in wrestling. His brain tumor revealed itself through an epileptic seizure, but otherwise he was perfectly healthy. His younger sister had died two years earlier of a malignant brain tumor that her doctor didn't even consider worth treating. His parents were desperate and ready to accept the worst. I removed a right frontal glioblastoma, the most malignant form of brain cancer.

After the operation, during long discussion, I convinced him and his parents that he should have radiotherapy. Now, more than fifteen years later, he is married, father of two lovely girls, enjoys life and works full-time. This course is rather unusual with such a malignant brain tumor. It does not really fit with the statistics; this patient is an exception.

The lesson I learned from this experience is that each patient should be given the chance to be such an exception whatever his or her prognosis, based on statistics, may be. The role of the neurosurgeon, besides technical skill and clinical competence, is to have enough psychological skill to convince the patient, when he or she is informed of the diagnosis, that there always is a chance to survive and that it is worthwhile fighting against the disease with all our energy. The patient and physician have to fight together, and this is only possible when a real human contact has been established between the two.

Chapter Five

Afterward: Never Underestimate Yourself

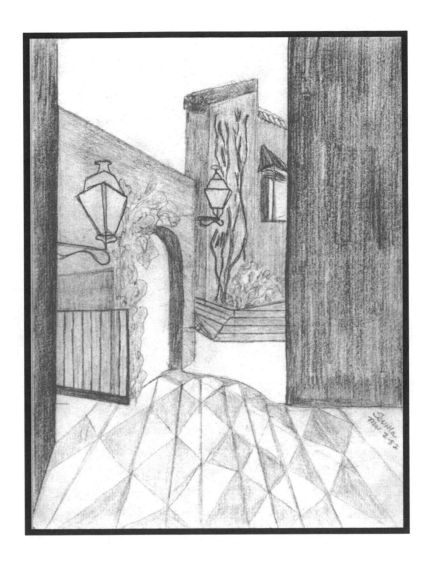

Never Underestimate Yourself

Afterward:

Never Underestimate Yourself

From beginning to end you will be taking small but courageous steps in learning about and dealing with the diagnosis, treatment and recovery afterwards. As one poet said, "We are like people climbing out of an immensely deep valley on a trail which only occasionally allows us glimpses of the geography below or the heights above." (Robert Gruden, The Art of Living)

Never forget that you yourself may be an inspiration to someone else. Those around you will be positively affected by your bravery in facing and dealing with your condition. Never underestimate your own internal resources; your own strengths; creative abilities; and common sense to handle this problem. Never underestimate the love of your friends and family. Asking friends and family for help gives them a gift: It gives them the opportunity to show you their love.

If you have lost a loved one, may these words by William Penn bring you some comfort: "They that love beyond the world cannot be separated by it. Death cannot kill what never dies. Nor can spirits ever be divided, that love and live in the same divine principle, the root and record of their friendship. Death is but crossing the world as friends do the seas; they live in one another. This is the comfort of friendship, that though they may be said to die, yet their friendship and society are, in the best sense, ever present because immortal."

No one is saying that this is an easy problem or that there are any magic solutions. Life presents us with many challenges that we didn't ask for. And yet, in them we must find our own meaning, and go forth. On behalf of all of the authors who shared their stories with you, we wish you a future filled with joy, prosperity, and good health.

—Your editor, Tricia

Part Three

Chapter Six

Resources

Navigating Through a Strange Land

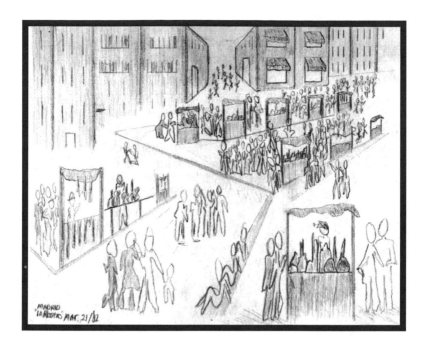

Resources

Decisions, Decisions, Decisions...

One of the most common themes of brain tumor patients is their bewilderment over often years of misdiagnosis, conflicting opinions from various specialists on the optimum treatment for their situation, and the confusing array of who, what, when, where, and how? It can be paralyzing trying to decide what to do or who to listen to.

Sometimes, it's clear cut; you just know the right thing to do. One patient knew from the start that she wasn't going to have surgery, even though she had an aggressive tumor. She has controlled it with a multitude of alternative therapies. Everyone is awed by her courage. She said of it, "I've just had this horrible gut feeling that if I go into surgery I won't come out alive." She is living by her gut instinct.

Choosing whether to have a particular surgery, radiation, chemotherapy, or whatever, is a personal decision that only you can make. You don't have to do any of it, if you don't want to. Some who have exhausted conventional treatment have opted for more controversial means. Even if this only allows for a few more months of life, if that time is of quality then no one else can place a judgement on that choice.

Navigating Through a Strange Land

Some people find facing their own mortality ultimately invigorating. There is a new found desire to live and live better than before. It strips away the pretentiousness. Life becomes full of meaning again—filled with a more personal meaning, not that imposed by others, or by society.

However, it's hard to fathom the difficulties that some people are faced with. Even though we as bystanders can learn something from and empathize with others sad tales, it is devastating to the people who have to live it. As one family member said, "My mother is going through hell, and there's no other way to say that." He says, "Think before rushing into something like radiation therapy."

Death, of course, is something that our society seems phobic about: No one will really talk about it. No one helps you to understand it as a child. Medical personnel view it is a failure, rather than a natural event. But death, like life, is a sacred event; we need to learn how to psychologically and spiritually prepare for death; so that it becomes welcomed, not feared. The hospice movement has been a savior to many families, as it does just this. But we all must help our own relatives and friends, when the end is near, to feel loved and honored for their contributions in life, so that they may go with peace on their face, not loneliness and sadness in their hearts.

Ultimately, the best way to relieve fear is through research, research, and research, because no one place will have all the answers. Research through libraries, physicians, friends, other patients, foundations, etc. You have to feel comfortable with the decisions you make. And once making a decision, decide that at the time that was your best choice. Don't wrack yourself with guilt if you find a different piece of information, such as a new procedure in Finland, later down the road. There's no such thing as the 'perfect decision,' just what makes sense at the time. The resources following will help you in the research process.

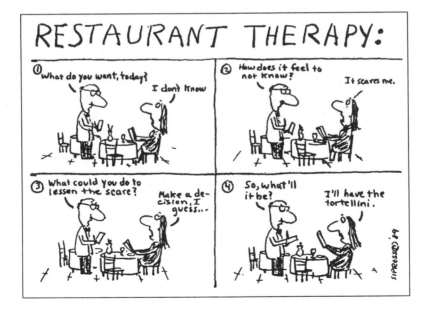

Navigating Through a Strange Land

Resources

Tumors and treatment

What to call it

In brief, a glossary of all but the most rare of tumors, treatments, and laboratory research.

Tumors

Astrocytomas (the most common primary brain tumor; graded by its aggressiveness)

Well-differentiated astrocytoma, low grade or grade I (slow growing)

Anaplastic astrocytoma, mid grade or grade II (cells more malignant, faster growing))

Glioblastoma multiforme, astrocytoma grade III (grow rapidly, cells are very malignant)

Acoustic neuroma (tumors of the cranial nerves, i.e. facial, hearing; very intricate area to operate on)

Brain stem glioma (means located at the base of the brain, cells range in type; usually affects children, 20% of childhood tumors)

Ependymoma (85% benign; usually localized and slow growing; but can be malignant)

Ganglioneuroma (slow growing, occurs in brain or spinal cord; most rare form of glioma)

Juvenile pilocytic astrocytoma (common childhood tumor; frequently occurs in the cerebellum; low grade, usually is easily cured)

Mixed glioma (mixed cells; treatment is based on the most malignant of the mix)

Oligodendroglioma (5% of all gliomas; relatively rare and is slow growing)

Resources

Optic nerve glioma (on or near nerves between the eye and brain vision centers; common in people who have neurofibromatosis; usually benign)

Chordoma (develop from spinal-like structure in fetal development; are slow growing)

Craniopharyngioma (near the pituitary; develop from left over cells in fetal development; usually affects infants and children; easily removed now)

Medulloblastoma (causes more than 25% of all childhood tumors; fast growing but responds well to treatment; located often in the cerebellum)

Meningioma (originates from the meninges, or lining of the brain and spinal cord; 15% of all brain tumors and 25% of all spinal cord tumors; is slow growing)

Pineal tumors (tumors that occur in the area of the pineal gland (up to 20 different kinds) deep within the brain; 1% of all brain tumors; many are benign and treatable)

Pituitary adenomas (10% of all tumors; occurs near the pituitary gland, the master gland of the body which secretes hormones that controls the body's other glands, regulating essential body processes) Tumor is defined by the hormones it secretes. Usually benign and easily treatable by microsurgery).

Prolactinoma: secretes prolactin (to produce milk).

Acromegaly: an effect of secreted growth hormone causing enlarged features such as hands, face.

Cushings disease: Outer shell of the adrenal glands secretes an excess of cortical hormones (ACTH). (In children, pituitary disturbances most commonly cause growth retardation, delayed puberty, diabetes insipidus, and Cushing's syndrome).

Primitive neuroectodermal tumors (several kinds; usually affects children and young adults; often very malignant and fast growing; spreads unevenly and is hard to remove entirely; surgery followed by high doses of radiation)

Schwannoma (cells around the nerve fibers; usually benign. aka. Acoustic Neuromas)

Vascular tumors (noncancerous, arising from blood vessels of the brain and spinal cord; easily treatable)

Treatments include

Surgery (microsurgery using the surgical microscope)

Radiation Therapy:

- Interstitial irradiation, also called Brachytherapy
- Radiosurgery, also called the Gamma Knife

Chemotherapy

- A combination of various drugs depending on the tumor.

Treatment for pituitary tumors include:

- Transphenoidal operation (through the upper lip and nasal passage).
- Bromocriptine (or Parlodel), in conjunction with surgery, or if surgery is not elected.
- Radiation, if surgery cannot remove entire tumor.

Current laboratory research for new treatments and/or cure are:

- Molecular biology: studying DNA for genetic causes
- Bromodeoxyuridine (BUdR): a drug used to tell how aggressive cells are.
- Polyamines: Chemicals in the body that help cause cell division, or growth; search is to find a drug that blocks these polyamines.
- Immunotherapy: stimulating the body's own immune response to kill cells.
- Boron Neuton Capture Therapy: getting tumor cells to absorb boron-10, then radiation and chemo will kill only those cells and not the normal cells.

Personal contact

If you would like to contact one of the authors of the personal stories, please call the National Brain Tumor Foundation's volunteer phone network. The foundation will contact them and give them your phone number. They would be happy to talk with you. That number is listed below.

Brain tumor foundations and associations

Money received from donations is used for research grants and services provided for your benefit such as information publications. While

Resources

they may sound like huge beaurocracies, most were started by a small group of people, or just one person, who wanted to give others like you what they didn't have during their own, or a relatives,illness. Each group has a slightly different focus; be it research fundraising, support services or written information, but each offer you something, especially a compassionate ear. I have listed them geographically.

An asterisk * means they are part of the North American Brain Tumor Coalition, a new informal network of groups who share resources and meet annually to see what else needs to be made available to the public, and how they can impact Washington, D.C. to increase dollars given to fund brain tumor research.

East coast

*The Brain Tumor Society, 60 Leo Birmingham Parkway, Boston, MA 02135-1116, Tel: (617) 783-0340, Fax: (617) 783-9217. Started in 1989. Publishes quarterly newsletter *Heads Up*; has support group information; a patient/family telephone network; and information on brain tumors. Holds an annual art auction, called Color Me Hope, to raise money. Contact Bonnie Feldman, founder, about donating your artwork for the auction.

*The Children's Brain Tumor Foundation, 35 Alpine Lane, Chappaqua, NY 10514, Tel: (914) 238-1656. Started in 1990 by 15 sets of parents. Has an annual all-day picnic in July for families. Holds its own support group which meets the last Thursday of the month in Manhatten, 7-9pm, at 19 E. 88 St., Suite 1D (at 5th Avenue). This is the one consistent group for the New York area. Has been meeting for 2 years. For information, call group leader Dr. Marsha Greenleaf at (212) 534-8877. Other activities mainly involve fundraising. Written patient information is referred to NBTF in San Francisco or ABTF in Chicago.

The Rainbow Foundation for Brain Tumor Research, Inc. ,P.O. Box 327 Highland Mills, NY 10930, Tel: (914) 928-8683. Started in 1990 by a husband and wife who lost their child in 1986. Holds annual Walkathon in October. Primarily fundraises (looking for volunteers!).

*The Brain Tumor Foundation for Children, Inc., 2231 Perimeter Park Drive, Suite 9, Atlanta, GA 30341, Tel: (404) 458-5554, Fax: (404) 458-5467. Started in 1984 by 11 parents. Publishes a newsletter approximately every 6 weeks which includes a column to answer medical questions by physicians. Formed a Teen Club to offer teenagers a source of support with their peers. They go golfing, picnicking, and whatever they decide on. Sponsors an annual golf tournament to raise money. Has a telephone network for patient support. Helps teenagers before going back to school with the "Transitional Learning Center" at Georgia State University. Is affiliated with Emory University and Egleston Children's Hospital for which it also raises funds (i.e. they funded a new pediatric research laboratory there).

Acoustic Neuroma Association, P.O. Box 12402, Atlanta, GA 30355, (404) 237-8023. Started in 1981. Targets benign cranionerve tumors including acoustic neuromas (eighth nerve tumors), meningiomas and other cranionerve tumors. Has booklets and pamphlets for patients. Has forty support groups around the country. Publishes quarterly newsletter, The Acoustic Neuroma Assocation Notes. Holds a bi-annual national symposium.

Ride for Kids Foundation, 6350 B McDonough Drive, Norcross, GA 30093. Tel: (404) 449-0789, Fax: (404) 449-9065. With sponsorships from the American Honda Motor Company and others, they organize local motorcycle groups to hold day long rides to raise money for research. Contact them for a listing of the upcoming bike rides around the country.

South

The South Florida Brain Tumor Association, P.O. Box 770182, Coral Springs, FL 33077-0182, Tel: (305) 748-4153. Started in 1991. Has organized two support groups in the area. Holds an annual conference in October on future research and treatment for health care professionals, patients and family, with noted national speakers.

Resources

Midwest

*American Brain Tumor Association, 2720 River Road, Suite 147, Des Plains, IL 60018, Tel: (708) 827-9910, Fax: (708) 827-9918. Publishes numerous detailed booklets on various aspects of brain tumor disease; has resource listings; information about support groups; social service referrals; CONNECTIONS—a pen pal program; and a listing of physicians who offer investigational treatments for brain tumors in adults and in children.

Brain Tumor Information Services, Box 405, Room J341, University of Chicago Hospitals, 5841 S. Maryland Avenue, Chicago, IL 60637, (312) 684-1400. Offers consultation and referrals to physicians who specialize in particular tumor types.

West

*National Brain Tumor Foundation, 785 Market Street, Suite 1600, San Francisco, CA 94103, Tel(s): 1(800) 934-CURE (2873) or (415) 284-0208 (Support line; hooks you up with other patients by phone), Fax: (415) 284-0209. Started in the early '80's as Friends of Brain Tumor Research. Publishes quarterly newsletter *Search;* a booklet listing all support groups in the U.S. and Canada; and *The Resource Guide* for patients and family (in-depth information). The first copy of these items are free. Holds bi-annual three day conference in San Francisco. Tapes are available for the talks given at the previous conference from CAL Tapes of Menlo Park, CA. Their number is 1-800-360-1145.

The Pituitary Tumor Network, 16350 Ventura Blvd. #231, Encino, CA 91436, Tel: (805) 499-9973, Fax: (805) 499-1523. Formed in 1993. Just published *The Pituitary Patient Resource Guide*, First Annual N. American Edition, a comprehensive reference book for pituitary patients, families, physicians, and health care providers. Lists particular physicians, centers, medications, financial assistance centers, home care specialists, publications, etc.

Navigating Through a Strange Land

Canada
*Brain Tumor Foundation of Canada, 111 Waterloo Street, Suite 600, London, Ontario N6B 2M4, Tel: (519) 642-7755, Fax: (519) 642-7192. Started in 1982 by a parent of an eight year old who succumbed to a brain tumor, and a neurosurgeon. Publishes the newsletter *Brainstorm* quarterly; the Adult Brain Tumor Patient Resource Handbook; the Pediatric Brain Tumor Handbook (for parents and teachers). Developed and maintains the Kelly Northey Memorial Library to provide educational materials to patients/families/physicians. Holds an annual information day in October. Is expanding a support group network across Canada and will help set up new ones for those interested in starting their own group.

Acoustic Neuroma Association of Canada, P.O. Box 369, Edmonton, Alberta T5J 2J6, Tel: (403) 428-3384; in Canada 1-800-561-2622 (ANAC). Started in 1984 by 4 patients. Publishes quarterly newsletter Connections; has booklets and video brochures; provides support, patient networking; and information on physio and facial neuromuscular rehabilitation and elleviation of post surgical problems.

Other services and information

Medical libraries

The National Library of Medicine, the world's largest research library is a resource for all U.S. health science libraries.MEDLARS (Medical Literature Analysis and Retrieval System) is a computerized system of more than 30 databases and databanks offered by the NLM. The on-line files are used by universities, medical schools and anyone interested in medical information. Databases include MEDLINE which cites international biomedical sources and DIRLINE, a directory of information resources, and others. Grateful Med is the program used to access it from a Macintosh^{TM} and modem. For more information on databases and how to access call the National Library of Medicine, MEDLARS Management Section (1-800-638-8480). Ask medical library staff if they can help show you how to use it. Some libraries charge an hourly fee.

Resources

For example, I asked for the subject category of Brain Tumors. I got 43 citations in the Magazine & Journal Articles category. I typed D 8 ABS to display the eighth citation's abstract:

8. Allen, Jeffrey C.
What we learn from infants with brain tumors. (Editorial)
New England Journal of Medicine v328, n24 (June 17, 1993); 1780 (2 pages). It then lists the summary of the article.

I also looked up brain tumors in the computerized book catalogue system at the medical library. There were 23 citations, mostly on treatment procedures. Another book to look in is the Books in Print, and Forthcoming Books in Print, in the reference section of the library. Looking under the topic heading of Brain Tumors, it will list all books in print and those coming out for the next season.

Consumer health information

Planetree of the California Pacific Medical Center of San Francisco is nationally known and highly respected for their library of consumer health information. Even if you do not live in the area, they can be an excellent source of health information and/or direction to specific publications and groups. They can compile an information packet on a specific topic or fax individual articles (nominal fee charged). Their number is (415) 923-3681.

Transportation, financial assistance, and equipment

American Cancer Society. Most chapters of the ACS will direct brain tumor inquiries for information to the brain tumor foundations already listed. However, other important services that they can provide are: 1) Local transportation; 2) Equipment, such as wheelchairs, canes, etc. 3) Emergency financial assistance; and 4) The Angel Flight Program, which offers help with commercial flights to treatments outside of your state. They will coordinate the flights. These services are provided through each chapter. Contact your local chapter.

Navigating Through a Strange Land

Medical consultation

Cancer Consultant Service (in San Francisco, call (415) 775-9956; or check with the American Cancer Society in your area to see if there is a similar service, or consult with the one in San Francisco.) Provides second opinions on diagnosis and treatment. An expert panel will look at medical records, biopsies, etc.

Written and verbal consultation on cancer

Physicians Data Query (PDQ). Provides information on current clinical research trials. Call with your exact tumor information and they will do a computer search and send you one free printout. Their number is (301) 496-7403.

National Cancer Institute. Through the National Institutes of Health, the NCI publishes excellent small self-help booklets. For example: "Radiation Therapy and You: A guide to self-help during treatment." The Cancer Information Service (CIS) of the NCI answers questions from the public. To get free single copies of their publications, or direct phone assistance, call (1-800-4-CANCER). They also just published a series of booklets on pain management after treatment, for clinicians and patients.

Neuroscience rehabilitation centers

Located around the country, these centers provide rehabilitation for head injuries, and usually includes services for brain tumor patients. Contact the neuroscience department of your local hospital to find where the closest one is. Or, contact the National Head Injury Foundation in Washington, D.C.

Brain tumor registries

The Central Brain Tumor Registry of the United States (CBTRUS), 3333 W. 47th St. Chicago, IL 60632. Phone: (312) 579-0021. The CBTRUS was established in July 1992 to provide a resource for gathering and disseminating statistical information on primary brain tumors, malignant and benign, to include brain, cranial nerve, meningial, spinal cord, pituitary and pineal neoplasms, so that the scientific community may utilize this data for the purposes of improved diagnosis, treatment, etiological studies and ultimately for the prevention of all brain tumors.

At present, they are collecting benign and malignant brain tumor data from 4 state registries and have contracted with 15 other state registries. Dr. Faith Davis, of the University of Illinois at Chicago, School of Public Health is the person conducting the study. If you are a patient with a malignant cancer you are automatically registered with the state registry. They encourage all registries to participate.

National Familial Brain Tumor Registry, The Johns Hopkins Oncology Center, 600 North Wolfe Street, Room 132, Baltimore, MD 21287-8936, (410) 955-0227. Researches family histories of brain tumors.

Cancer retreats, alternative therapies, and hospices
Commonweal is a well known retreat for people with cancer on the West Coast. The founder of Commonweal, Michael Lerner, has a new book out titled: *Choices in Healing: Integrating the Best of Conventional and Complimentary Approaches to Cancer.* 628 pages of the most current information on cancer therapies and alternate healing practices. Published by MIT Press. Their number is (415) 868-0970. There may be something like this in your area.

The Wellness Community in Santa Monica, CA has been around for about 20 years. They focus on alternative healing practices and therapies. Harold Benjamin, Ph.D. one of the founders wrote the book *The Wellness Community Guide to Fighting for Recovery: From Victim to Victor.* Their number is (310) 314-2555.

National Hospice Association, Arlington, VA, (703) 243-5900. Hospice provides specialized services and assistance to the terminally ill and/or dying patient and their caregivers. Includes nursing, counseling and volunteer services. Call the national association for a hospice near you.

Navigating Through a Strange Land

Beauty aids

Knight and Day Hair Products, Inc., P.O. Box 849, Corte Madera, CA 94925, (415) 381-8018. Specializing in customized wigs and services for total or partial hair loss.

Designs for Comfort, Inc., P.O. Box 8229, Northfield, IL 60093, 1-800-621-5839. Designs a combination cap and hairpiece called the "head-liner," an alternative to a wig.

Therapists

Ask the hospital social worker or clinic staff for referrals to reputable and well-liked counselors. Some may be on staff at the same hospital. Or, call the local chapters of the professional associations for a listing of therapists in your area. Look through your local telephone directory. For example, under psychotherapists in the yellow pages is listed the "San Francisco Psychological Association: the official chapter of the California Psychological Association." They provide free information and referrals to match your specific needs with the right therapist. Check your directory for this kind of comprehensive group. And, check with friends.

Ask the hospital about their chaplain services, or your local church adminstrators about pastors, reverends, rabbi's and other church clergy who you can talk with.

Creativity and the arts

Artistic pursuits: Art and writing are very therapeutic tools to express our innermost needs and wants. This may include keeping a daily journal of thoughts, feelings, desires, conflicts; writing poetry or short stories; keeping a dream journal; drawing, painting, pottery, or anything that helps to communicate on a different level. Check with the local community college for classes on creative writing and other arts. There are also retreats specifically for writing. Ask the college English Department about these kinds of programs.

Resources

Legal and financial planning

Disability, job discrimination and insurance

The National Coalition for Cancer Survivorship (NCCS) will help you with discrimination either in your job or with insurance companies. They can be reached at (301) 585-2616. Publishes *What cancer survivors need to know about health insurance,* by Irene C. Card, of the NCCS.

The National Organization on Disability in Washington D.C. can help you with issues of how to file for benefits, who qualifies, what's necessary, discrimination, etc. Their number is (202) 293-5960.

Your city and state **Social Security Administration listed in the phone book under government offices** is the office you contact for state disability insurance claims. Call them to get detailed information on the procedure.

The American Association of Retired Persons (AARP) has a wealth of information on retirement issues. Could be important information for people who retire on a disability income. Call your local chapter to find out more information about their services and if they can help you. National headquarters is at 1909 K St. NW, Washington D.C. 20049, tel: (202) 872-4700.

AARP Widowed Persons Service can help with financial advice. Their number is (202) 434-2260. Newly widowed persons should also make an appointment with the Social Security office to claim their spouse's benefit. As a widower you're entitled to 100% of the benefit after the age of 65 and a reduced benefit after 60, or at any age if you have children living with you.

The Information and Referral (I and R) program can direct you to Help Agencies. Contact your local **United Way** for information.

Navigating Through a Strange Land

Financial planners

Institute of Certified Financial Planners (ICFP), 600 E. Eastman Ave., Ste. 301, Denver, CO 80231-4397, 1-800-322-4237 (information services). 7,200 CFP's nationwide work full-time at financial planning. This organization will give you a listing of planners by area.

National Association of Personal Financial Advisors, 1130 Lake Cook Rd., Ste. 105, Buffalo Grove, IL, 1-800-366-2732. A small group of 'fee only' planners. They will send you a listing of full time planners in your area.

Choices in Dying, 250 West 57th St. , New York, NY 10107, Tel: (212) 246-6973. Non-profit group that provides information and current forms for living wills and durable powers of attorney for health care.

Legal computer software

Willmaker 5: Focuses on wills, living wills and final arrangements documents. Discusses federal and state estate taxes and proxy requirements for health care directives. Published by Nolo Press
For DOS 3.0; Windows 3.1 or Mac 6.0.4. 800-992-6656, $69.00

It's Legal 4.0: It's Legal contains 41 documents. Includes business planning, home buying, corporate documents for boards of directors, a memorial service planning worksheet and living trust documents.
For DOS and Windows 3.1. 1-800-223-6925 $49.00

Home Lawyer 2.0: 16 legal documents compiled by Joel Hyatt of Hyatt Legal Services. Among other general documents it includes a will and living will, general and medical powers of attorney. DOS 2.1 or later systems. 1-800-820-7458, $69.95

Personal Law Firm 2.0: Personal Law Firm has more documents than Home Lawyer but are more aimed at business and marital issues. Browsing or calling the company before buying is recommended. For DOS 3.3 or greater. (415) 454-7101, $99.00

Resources

Reading list

I have picked books that I have either read myself or were recommended to me, or that looked good, inspiring or non-threatening on the bookshelf.

Brain tumors and neurologically related books

As you may already have found out there aren't many books on this subject. Since it seems to be an area that could use a few more books, maybe you yourself will write the next one!

Gifts of Time, Dr. Fred Epstein, Pediatric Neurosurgeon, William Morrow, 1993: Tracks stories of children with brain tumors

Death Be Not Proud, John Gunther, Harper, 1989: Memoir of a boy's struggle with a brain tumor, written by his father.

Alex's Journey, American Brain Tumor Association: Story of a child with a brain tumor; written for children to understand the process, contact them directly at address above.

Brain Tumors: A Monograph, Dr. Stephen R. Freidberg, Chairman of Neurosurgery at the Lahey Clinic Foundation, Burlington, Mass., published by Ciba-Geigy Pharmaceutical Co., vol. 38, 32 pages. Last revised 1986.

The Human Brain, Its Functions and Capabilities, Isaac Asimov, New American Library. :For a general understanding of how the brain works.

Neuro—Life on the Frontlines of Brain Surgery and Neurological Medicine, David Noonan, Ivy Books, 1989

Cancer books

Alternatives in Cancer Therapy, Ross Pelton, R.Ph., Ph.D., and Lee Overholser, Ph.D., Simon and Schuster, 1994:Analyzes controversial alternative therapies.

Cancervive: The Challenge of Life After Cancer, Susan Nessim and Judith Ellis Houghton Mifflin, 1991

Everyone's Guide to Cancer Therapy, Malin Dollinger, MD, Ernest H. Rosenbaum, MD, and Greg Cable, Andrews & McNeal publishers, 1991

Navigating Through a Strange Land

Coping with Chemotherapy, Nancy Bruning, Ballantine Books, 1993
Spontaneous Remission: An Annotated Bibliography, Brendan O'Regan and Caryle Hirshberg, Institute of Noetic Sciences, 1993, 475 Gate Five Rd., Sausalito, CA 94965: The world's largest electronic database of medically reported cases of spontaneous remission of cancer and other diseases. A tome written for medical researchers, but inquisitive cancer patients will be fascinated by it, says the NCCS newsletter's book reviewer.

For women
Beauty and Cancer, Diane Doan Noyes, Peggy Mellody, R.N., AC Press, Los Angeles, 1988
Color Me Beautiful, Carole Jackson, Ballantine Books, 1980

On death, loss and recovery
The story of Jamie was from: *To Live Until We Say Goodbye*, Elisabeth Kubler Ross and Mal Warshaw, Prentice-Hall, 1978: Essays and photographs of people in their final stages. Other books by Dr. Ross are: *On Death and Dying*, 1969 ; *Living with Death and Dying*, 1981; *On Children and Death*, 1983; *Death*, 1975; *Questions and Answers on Death and Dying*, 1974
Losing A Parent: Passage to New Way of Living, Alexandra Kennedy, Harper-Collins, 1991
How It Feels When a Parent Dies, Jill Krementz, Alfred A. Knopf, 1991:Children tell their own stories of a parents death
Utne Reader (The best of the alternative press) "Facing Death: It's inevitable, it's difficult, and it just might transform your life." No. 47, Sept./ Oct. 1991, pages 65-88. Call (612) 338-5040 to find out how to get a back copy.
Necessary Losses, Judith Viorst, Ph.D., Fawcett, 1988
Living Through A Personal Crisis, Ann Kaiser Stearns, 1984, Ballantine Books reprint, 1988: Hospital chaplain explains crisis and feelings of loss
Coming Back, Ann Kaiser-Stearns, Ballantine Books, 1988 (a follow up to her previous book).
Living Through Loss: God's Help in Bereavement, David Winter,Shaw Pubs., 1986

Resources

Anatomy of An Illness, As Perceived by the Patient, Norman Cousins, 1979 reprint by W.W. Norton & Co., 1987

The Healing Family (The Simonton Approach for Families facing Illness). Stephanie Matthews Simonton, Bantam Books, 1984. Provides help for maintaining the family in times of crisis.

Building a New Dream: A Family Guide to Coping with Chronic Illness and Disability, Janet R. Maurer, MD and Patricia D. Strasberg, Ed.D, 1989

Living With Chronic Illness: Days of Patience and Passion, Cheri Register, Free Press, 1989

We Are Not Alone: Learning to Live with Chronic Illness, Sefra Pitzele, Workman Publishing, 1986

Creativity, inspiration, poetry

The Prophet, Kahlil Gibran, Alfred A. Knopf, Inc., 1923

Gathering of Hope, Helen Hayes, Walker & Co.1989

The Grace of Great Things—Creativity and Innovation, Robert Grudin, Tickner & Fields, 1990

The Art of Living, Robert Grudin, Tickner & Fields, 1988: Elegant philosophies on life by an English professor

The Creative Spirit, Daniel Goleman, Paul Kaufman and Michael Ray: Based on the PBS television series. Penguin Books, 1992: Encourages reevaluation of innate creativity without judgement.

Creativity and Madness: Psychological Studies of Art and Artists, Barry Panter, MD, PhD and Bernie Virshup, MD, 1994, Published by the American Institute of Medical Education (AIMED) 2625 W. Alemeda Ave. Ste. 504, Burbank, CA 91905, 1-800-348-8441: Provides insights into the lives and works of the world's greatest artists. This group also holds 2 annual meetings for health care professionals.

The Tao of Inner Peace, Diane Dreher, Harper-Perennial, 1991

Everyday Zen in Love and Work, Charlotte Joko Beck, Harper & Row, 1989

Ecstacy, Understanding the Psychology of Joy, Robert A. Johnson, Harper-Collins, 1987

Living a Balanced Life: Applying Timeless Spiritual Teachings to Your Everyday Life, Eliott James, Dhamma Books, 1990

Living a Beautiful Life: Five Hundred Ways to Add Elegence, Order, Beauty and Joy to Every Day of Your Life, Alexandra Stoddard, Avon Books, 1988
Taming Your Gremlin: A Guide to Enjoying Yourself, Richard Carson, Harper-Collins 1983

Money
Your Money or Your Life, Vicki Robin and Joe Dominguez, Viking Penquin Book, Inc., 1992: A great book on work, money and security.

Catalogue book services/specialty publishers
Legal
Nolo Press, a self-help legal publishing company in Berkeley, CA., publishes titles such as: *Plan Your Estate With a Living Trust; Nolo's Simple Will Book; Who Will Handle Your Finances if You Can't; The Conservatorship Book; How to Probate an Estate;* and others. Has software also. Consult the company for a brochure. Their number is (510) 549-1976, Address: 950 Parker Street, Berkeley, CA 94710-9867

Mind/body medicine
The Institute for the Study of Human Knowledge, run by David S. Sobel, MD, and Robert Ornstein, MD, who wrote *The Healing Brain*, have a book/tape service, called Mental Medicine, of the most current books on mind/body medicine. Write to: ISHK Book Service, Dept. C19M, P.O. Box 176, Los Altos, CA 94023 to be put on mailing list. They also publish a newsletter called Mental Medicine Update, for $9.95 yearly subscription.
The Association for Research and Enlightenment: A-R-E Press: A catalogue of new age books and videos, P.O. Box 656, 68th St. and Atlantic Avenue, VA 23451-0656, or 1-800-723-1112.

Psychology
Sterns Book Service mail order house and store (Important and readable books in the fields of psychology, therapy and human potential). (312) 769-4460. For example: "Behind The Family Mask: Therapeutic Change

in Rigid Family Systems; Midnight Musings of a Family Therapist; Black Sheep and Kissing Cousins: How our Family Stories Affect Us. Academic but readable.

Art therapy

Brunner/Mazel Publishers, 19 Union Square West, New York, NY 10003, (212) 924-3344: Publishes books on Art Therapy by clinicians who pioneered the field. Titles such as Clinical Art Therapy; Family Art Psychotherapy; Adolescent Art Therapy; Adult Art Psychotherapy. Fascinating work being done in collaboration with the medical profession.

I'm sure there are a zillion books that are wonderful, but there's only so much time in the day. The bookstore kept shooing me out at 5:00pm.

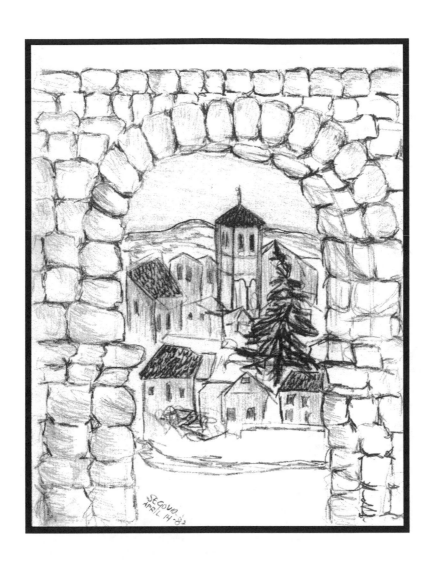

Index

A

Ammenorria, 99
Anger, 117, 185
Arlinghaus, Julie, 76
Art therapy, 54, 109-110, 118, 222
Astrocytoma, 72, 76, 143

B

Beckerman, Marie, 40
Bibel, Debra Jan, 188
Brain tumors
  in child, 115
  in adolescent/young adult, 25,
  29, 44, 76, 81, 99, 122, 140
  in adult, 38, 63, 67, 132, 143,
  177
  Diagnosis of, 5
  Statistics of, 6
  Types of, 6-7, 212-213
  Philosophy of, 8
  Psychological aspects, 159
  Progression of, 8-9
  Treatment of, 9
Broyard, Anatole, 155
Brueggemann, Walter, 187
Buchholz, William, 189

C

Coalition, 129
Coping
  control, 159
  faith, 177
  hope, 189
  pets, 164
  unable to, 147
  with death, 187, 203, 210
  Zen, 188
Craniotomy, 88
Craniopharyngioma, 44

D

Death
  of child, 115
  of adolescent, 122,198
  of parent/spouse, 132, 177
De Jong, Chris, 81
De Tribolet, Nicholas, 198
Decadron, 123
Dilantin, 30
Disability
  going on, 63
Disraeli, 89
Dostoevski, 94

F

Family structure, 184
Farbach, Peter, 13
Feldman, Bonnie, 122
Feldman, Seth, 122
Fifth cranial nerve, 38
Fiore, Margaret, 13
Forstner, Darryl, 132
Frankl, Victor, 96

G

Ganglioneuroma, 29,140
Gladson, Karyn, 177
Glioblastoma, 25, 63, 81, 122, 132,
  177, 198
Grief, 108
Gruden, Robert, 203

H

Hail, Richard, 140
Hydroxeurea, 91

I

Impairment
  language, 171
  physical, 145

H
Headaches, 25, 82
Hospice, 210
Hydrocephalus, 173
J
Juvenile Pilocytic Astrocytoma, 76
K
Kornsand, Norman, 63
Kubler-Ross, Elizabeth, 115, 160
Kuchera, Chris, 72
L
Lamb, Sharon, 12
M
Memory
    problems with, 169
Meningioma, 38, 67
M.O.P.P., 124
N
Necrosis, 63, 146
Neuropsychology, 167
    testing, 173
P
Pain, 39, 47, 83, 146, 185
Paralysis, 145, 186
Penn, William, 203
Pituitary Adenoma, 99
Professionals/care
    coordinating care, 10, 137, 199
    estate planning, 11
    neuroscience nurses, 12
    social workers, 14
    chaplains, 14
    neuropsychologist, 14
    marriage and family therapist, 15
    support groups, 17
Prolactin, 100

Psychoanalysis, 155
R
Realistic hopefulness, 175
Research
    importance of, 210
Rhizotomy, 39
Roloff, Tricia, 99
RU-486, 67
S
Santi, Laura, 29
Sapowski, Robert, 161
Seed implants, 63
Seizures
    frequent, 148
    petit mal, 73
    psychomotor, 29
Self-transcendence, 157
Siegel, Bernie, 28, 86, 162
Simonsen, Kris, 44
Smith, Harry, 143
Spiegel, David, 86, 163
Spontaneous remission, 162
Stroke, 148
T
Talmud, 98
Tegretol, 41
Transphenoidal, 44,
Takano, Fume, 67
U
Ubuntu, 95
V
Vertigo, 39
W
Walcott, 94
Walker, John, 167
Wilson, Charles, 159

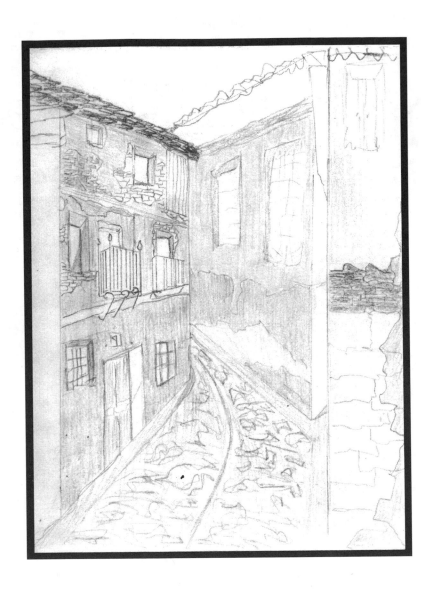